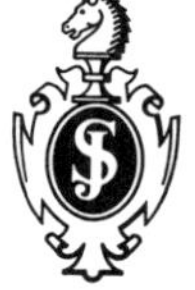

E&M Endocrinology and Metabolism

Progress in Research and Clinical Practice

Margo Panush Cohen   Piero P. Foà

Series Editors

Endocrinology and Metabolism
Progress in Research and Clinical Practice

Margo Panush Cohen   Piero P. Foà
  Series Editors

Cohen and Foà (eds): Hormone Resistance and Other Endocrine Paradoxes
  (Vol. 1)

Jovanovic (ed.): Controversies in Diabetes and Pregnancy (Vol. 2)

Forthcoming volumes:

Cohen and Foà (eds.): The Brain as an Endocrine Organ (Vol. 3)

Ginsberg-Fellner and McEvoy (eds): Autoimmunity and the Pathogenesis of
  Diabetes (Vol. 4)

Lois Jovanovic
Editor

Controversies in Diabetes and Pregnancy

With a Foreword by Steven G. Gabbe

With 36 Illustrations, 4 in Full Color

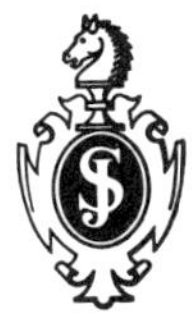

Springer-Verlag
New York Berlin Heidelberg
London Paris Tokyo

Lois Jovanovic, M.D.
Senior Scientist
Sansum Medical Research Foundation
Santa Barbara, CA 93105
USA

Series Editors

Margo Panush Cohen, M.D., Ph.D.
Professor of Medicine
University of Medicine and
  Dentistry of New Jersey
Newark, NJ 07103
Director, Institute for Metabolic
  Research
University City Science Center
Philadelphia, PA 19104
USA

Piero P. Foà, M.D., Sc.D.
Professor Emeritus of Physiology
Wayne State University
Chairman Emeritus
Department of Research
Sinai Hospital
Detroit, MI
Mailing address:
  2104 Rhine Road
  West Bloomfield, MI 48033
  USA

Library of Congress Cataloging-in-Publication Data
Controversies in diabetes and pregnancy.
  (Endrocrinology and metabolism ; v. 2)
  1. Diabetes in pregnancy. I. Jovanovic, Lois.
II. Series. [DNLM: 1. Pregnancy in Diabetes.
WQ 248 C764]
RG580.D5C66   1988   618.3'26   87-28485

Typeset by David E. Seham Associates Inc., Metuchen, New Jersey.
Printed and bound by Arcata Graphics/Halliday, West Hanover, Massachusetts.
Printed in the United States of America.

9 8 7 6 5 4 3 2 1

ISBN 0-387-96622-6   Springer-Verlag New York Berlin Heidelberg
ISBN 3-540-96622-6   Springer-Verlag Berlin Heidelberg New York

Foreword

As I read this unique volume on diabetes and pregnancy edited by Lois Jovanovic, I was struck by two themes that run throughout these collected chapters. First, this volume provides an excellent assessment of past problems, present management, and future challenges presented by diabetes in pregnancy. Drury's unique, longitudinal experience with diabetes in pregnancy provides the reader with an important overview, as does Coetzee's discussion of gestational diabetes. Current problems—determining the etiology and prevention of congenital malformations in infants of diabetic mothers (IDM), assessment of antepartum fetal condition, management of pregnant patients with diabetic retinopathy, recognition of thyroid dysfunction in the pregnant diabetic woman, and understanding the multitude of metabolic sequelae observed in the IDM—are thoroughly reviewed. Finally, important considerations for future treatment and therapy such as the adaptation of the fetal pancreas to the disordered intrauterine environment often seen in maternal diabetes, the use of fetal pancreatic tissue for transplantation, the application of exercise in the management of the pregnant woman with diabetes, and the long-term consequences for the IDM provide an exciting glimpse into the future.

The second important theme that emerges is the critical role the problem of diabetes in pregnancy has played in our understanding of maternal and fetal physiology. Clinical observations supported by basic research have emphasized the role of fetal fuels in teratogenesis. Studies of both the macrosomic infant and the hyperinsulinemic animal model have demonstrated the importance of insulin as a fetal growth hormone. Our understanding of normal surfactant synthesis and of the effects of hyperglycemia and hyperinsulinemia has been enhanced by studies of the IDM. The impact pregnancy may have on diabetic retinopathy may prove important in our understanding of this complication in nonpregnant patients. I am certain that further investigations into the effects of diabetes on pregnancy and pregnancy on diabetes will yield significant findings.

With these thoughts in mind, I hope that as the reader enjoys each of these excellent contributions, he or she will find that the whole can be greater than the sum of its parts.

Columbus, Ohio

Steven G. Gabbe, M.D.
Professor and Chairman
Department of Obstetrics
  and Gynecology
The Ohio State University
  College of Medicine

Preface

It is a great honor to be the editor of this volume, *Controversies in Diabetes and Pregnancy,* for these collected works not only represent "state of the art" information, but also serve as a forum for the expression of opinion; in many cases it may even be the minority opinion. To fully enjoy this book, the reader should have a basic understanding of the field of diabetes and pregnancy. In this sense, the book is for the serious student of the topic of pregnancy and glucose metabolism.

A basic theme that unites all the works in this volume is the philosophy that normalization of maternal blood glucose throughout pregnancy will normalize the outcome of such pregnancies. Even this basic tenet is controversial in some circles. But the book also discusses minor themes that have become contested issues, such as the utility of exercise as a treatment modality for glucose intolerance in pregnancy, and the management and timing of delivery. Because each author assumed that the reader would be familiar with basic approaches and definitions, many chapters begin with the debate. Although in one chapter the author redefines the terminology of gestational diabetes, he does not do this for the naive reader, but he does it to have definitions conform with his views about treatment modalities. Several of the approaches incorporate agents that currently are not approved for use during pregnancy in the United States. The section on the use of oral hypoglycemic agents for the treatment of the gestational diabetic woman is particularly interesting for the American reader, who may learn from this large series that there might be a better way. In addition, a closely observed group of women in good glucose control were given the "ticket to go to term" without the "benefit" of fetal surveillance protocols. Here, too, there is a take-home message.

The section on fetal islet ontogeny contains an essay on the impact of maternal fuels on the development of the fetal pancreas. Then comes a chapter that deals with the delicate subject of the use of fetal tissue for transplantation in persons with diabetes. Both chapters suggest the possibility that there may someday be a cure for a disease that afflicts more than 17 million persons.

In addition to presenting pathophysiology and alternative treatment protocols, this work also provides a glimpse at the fetus in diabetic pregnancy. There is a chapter on the immediate neonatal metabolic picture and a chapter on the long-term follow-up of infants of diabetic mothers. These two chapters allow readers to form their own opinion on whether normalization of maternal blood glucose is worth all the time, effort, and expense if the infant outcome is the variable of interest.

Although this work does not pretend to be a comprehensive review of the entire field of diabetes and pregnancy, each chapter is well-annotated to allow for more reading.

I hope you will enjoy and profit from these collected works written with fervor, assertion, and sometimes pure faith, about a very exciting and controversial field.

Santa Barbara, California   Lois Jovanovic, M.D.

Contents

Part IV   Obstetrics Management

Part V   Infant Outcome of Pregnancies Complicated by Diabetes

Contributors

Raul Artal, M.D.
Associate Professor of Obstetrics and Gynecology, Department of Obstetrics and Gynecology, University of Southern California, Los Angeles, California, USA

Peter H. Bennett, M.B., F.R.C.P., F.F.C.M.
Chief, Phoenix Epidemiology and Clinical Research Branch, National Institute of Diabetes, Digestive and Kidney Diseases, Phoenix, Arizona, USA

Luis A. Bracero, M.D.
Assistant Professor, Department of Obstetrics and Gynecology, New York Medical College, Valhalla, New York, USA

Edward J. Coetzee, M.D.
Senior Lecturer and Specialist, Department of Obstetrics and Gynecology; Head, Ultrasound Diagnosis (Obstetrics and Gynecology), Obstetric Diabetic Service, Postgraduate Lecture Program, Medical School, University of Cape Town, Observatory, Cape Province, Republic of South Africa

Richard M. Cowett, M.D.
Associate Professor of Pediatrics, Brown University; Physician-in-Charge of the Special Care Nursery, Women and Infants Hospital of Rhode Island, Providence, Rhode Island, USA

M.I. Drury, M.D., F.R.C.P.I., F.R.C.O.G., D.Sc., (Q.U.B. Hon.), F.A.C.P. (Hon.)
Professor (acting) of Therapeutics, University College Dublin; Physician/Endocrinologist, Mater Misericordiae Hospital, National Maternity Hospital, Coombe-Lying-In-Hospital, Rotunda Hospital, Dublin, Ireland

Ulf J. Eriksson, M.D., Ph.D.
Associate Professor, Department of Medical Cell Biology, Uppsala University School of Medicine, Uppsala, Sweden

PIERO P. FOÀ, M.D., Sc.D.
Professor Emeritus of Physiology, Wayne State University; Chairman Emeritus, Department of Research, Sinai Hospital, Detroit, Michigan; Mailing address: 2104 Rhine Road, West Bloomfield, Michigan 48033, USA

BENT FORMBY, PH.D., D. Sc.
Senior Biochemist, Sansum Medical Research Foundation, Santa Barbara, California, USA

W.P.U. JACKSON, M.D.
Professor-Emeritus, Department of Medicine, University of Cape Town; Former Head of Endocrinology and Diabetes, University of Cape Town Teaching Hospital, Observatory, Cape Province, Republic of South Africa

LOIS JOVANOVIC, M.D.
Senior Scientist, Sansum Medical Research Foundation, Santa Barbara, California, USA

BARBARA E.K. KLEIN, M.D., M.P.H.
Associate Professor of Ophthalmology, University of Wisconsin School of Medicine, Madison, Wisconsin, USA

CHARLES M. PETERSON, M.D.
Director of Research, Sansum Medical Research Foundation, Santa Barbara, California, USA

DAVID J. PETTITT, M.D.
Assistant Chief, Diabetes and Arthritis Epidemiology Section, Phoenix Epidemiology and Clinical Research Branch, National Institute of Diabetes, Digestive and Kidney Diseases, Phoenix, Arizona, USA

HAROLD SCHULMAN, M.D.
Professor of Obstetrics and Gynecology, State University of New York at Stony Brook, Stony Brook, New York; Chairman, Department of Obstetrics and Gynecology, Winthrop-University Hospital, Mineola, New York, USA

KATHRYN R. SLAINE, M.D.
Medical Staff Fellow, National Institute of Health, Phoenix, Arizona, USA

Part I   Animal Models for the Study of Diabetes and Pregnancy

1
Experimental Studies of Congenital Malformations in Diabetic Pregnancy

Ulf J. Eriksson

Introduction

Despite considerable progress in the clinical management of diabetic pregnancy, the incidence of congenital malformations is approximately three times greater in infants of diabetic mothers than in the offspring of nondiabetic women (1–6). Congenital malformations observed in the infants of diabetic mothers more often tend to be multiple, more severe, and lethal than those seen in infants of nondiabetic mothers (3,5,6). The incidence of congenital malformations has not changed over the last few decades, whereas that of almost all other complications has decreased (4). The relative importance of malformations has therefore increased, and they are presently the most common cause of perinatal death among infants of diabetic mothers (5).

The etiology of the disturbance in embryo-fetal development in diabetic pregnancy is unclear. A number of studies have been carried out on different animal models with the aim of uncovering disruptive mechanisms that also may be operative in human diabetic pregnancy. This chapter reviews experimental results concerning disturbed development during pregnancy complicated by maternal diabetes or diabetes-like conditions, giving special attention to possible teratologic mechanisms. In this context, one particular aspect of altered embryo-fetal development in diabetic pregnancy, the somatic growth of the offspring, is noteworthy. The demonstration of accelerated fetal growth in late human diabetic pregnancy (3), and of growth delay in early human (7) and rat (8) diabetic pregnancy, has led several investigators to propose that growth retardation has a role in human teratogenesis (7,9,10). Nevertheless, research on fetal malformations in experimental animals is scant. The world literature concerning malformed offspring of diabetic animals consists of only about 30 papers (Tables 1.1a and 1.1b), and the number of studies of disturbed fetal development during other diabetes-associated conditions in vivo is slightly less (Table 1.2). There have also been a few in vitro studies of disturbed embryologic development during diabetes-like conditions, mainly with use of the whole-embryo culture technique (Table 1.3).

Maternal Diabetes

The first studies of malformations in the offspring of diabetic animals were undertaken more than 30 years ago in mice and rats that were made diabetic with alloxan after conception (11–13). In an early report, Fujimoto and collaborators described fetal anomalies and resorptions induced by alloxan treatment of pregnant rabbits (14). These findings were corroborated in a later study of alloxan-diabetic rabbit pregnancies in which increased fetal mortality and disturbed brain development were observed among the offspring (18). Although the diabetogenic drug was administered at various times both before and during pregnancy, malformations were observed only when it was injected on gestational days 2 and 9. Most of the studies reported during the 1960s and early 1970s used alloxan-diabetic mice (Table 1.1a), and eye anomalies, skeletal malformations, and increased mortality were the notable findings in the fetuses of these mice (15,16,19,21,22).

In 1966 Endo published the first report (in English) on a study in which all the experimental animals were made diabetic before the onset of pregnancy (19). He noted skeletal malformations in the offspring and an increased stillbirth rate. In the same year, the first investigation showing a beneficial effect of insulin treatment during pregnancy was published, indicating that the incidence of malformations dropped to normal levels in offspring of insulin-treated diabetic mice and that the proportion of unsuccessful pregnancies also decreased in these mice (20). Subsequently, Ichikari found that administration of tolbutamide to mice that were made alloxan-diabetic on gestational day 10 reduced the incidence of fetal malformations among their offspring to normal levels (23). These results are especially intriguing in view of the recent report that the predominant teratogenic period in rodents is before gestational day 10 (see below).

Examining the effects of alloxan injected into mice and rats on gestational days 0 and 7, Takano and Nishimura found a 50% malformation rate in the offspring of the diabetic mice, where external malformations were visually noted, and internal malformations were detected by whole-body transverse sectioning and alizarin red staining (21). Diabetic rats and mice also had an increased number of dead and resorbed fetuses. Deuchar observed an increased incidence of brain and heart abnormalities in mid-gestational embryos of alloxan- and streptozotocin(SZ)-diabetic rats that had been rendered diabetic during and before pregnancy (28). On gestational day 20, the offspring of SZ-diabetic rats showed an increased incidence of several different types of fetal malformations. Regardless of gestational age, the incidence of dead offspring was higher in the diabetic groups.

TABLE 1.1a. Congenital malformations (CM) in offspring of experimentally diabetic animals.

Reference	Year	Animal	Drug	Day of drug injection	Type of diabetes	Day of study	CM (%)	Type of CM
Ross and Spector (11)	1952	Mouse	Alloxan	Day 0–3	SD	18	29	Various
Bartelheimer and Kloos (12)	1952	Rat	Alloxan	Day 2–18	SD–MD	NB	7	Eye, tail
Kreshover et al (13)	1953	Rat	Alloxan	Day 0–20	SD	NB–PP	—	Dental
Fujimoto et al (14)	1958	Rabbit	Alloxan	Before pregnancy	SD–MD	15–31	46	Eye, skeletal, CNS
Koskenoja (15)	1961	Mouse	Alloxan	Before pregnancy	SD–MD	PP	8	Eye
Watanabe and Ingalls (16)	1963	Mouse	Alloxan	Day 8–13	MD	18	10	Skeletal
Mohr et al (17)	1964	Rat	Alloxan	Day 10	MD	14–22	—	Placental
Barashev (18)	1965	Rabbit	Alloxan	Before pregnancy or day 2–24	SD–MD	24–30	3	Brain
Endo (19)	1966	Mouse	Alloxan	Before pregnancy	MD	18	8	Skeletal
Horii et al (20)	1966	Mouse	Alloxan	Day 3	MD	18	5	CNS, eye, skeletal
		Mouse	Alloxan	Day 3	MDI	18	0.2	Cleft palate
Takano and Nishimura (21)	1967	Mouse	Alloxan	Day 0	MD	18	7	CNS, skeletal
		Rat	SZ	Day 7	MD	20	50	CNS, eye, skeletal
Endo and Ingalls (22)	1968	Mouse	Alloxan	Before pregnancy	MD	18	3	Skeletal
		Mouse	Alloxan	Before pregnancy	MD	18	16	Chromosomal breaks
Ichikari (23)	1970	Mouse	Alloxan	Day 9	SD	18	3	Skeletal, omphalocele
		Mouse	Alloxan	Day 9	SDT	18	0.2	Skeletal
Yamamoto et al (24)	1971	Mouse	Alloxan	Before pregnancy	MD	3	25–32	Chromosomal breaks

Abbreviations: SD = subdiabetic (mildly diabetic) animals, SDT = SD and tolbutamide treated, MD = manifest (severely) diabetic animals, MDI = MD and insulin treated, NB = newborn, PP = postpartum, SZ = streptozotocin.

TABLE 1.1b. Congenital malformations (CM) in offspring of spontaneously and experimentally diabetic animals.

Reference	Year	Animal	Drug	Day of drug injection	Type of diabetes	Day of study	CM (%)	Type of CM
Prager et al (25)	1974	Rat	SZ	Before pregnancy	MD	20	50	Placental cysts
Emmrich and Caffier (26)	1976	Rat	SZ	Day 4	MD	17–20	22	Placental cysts
Liban et al (27)	1976	Rat	SZ	Before pregnancy	MD	day 20	—	Placental cysts
Deuchar (28)	1977	Rat	Alloxan	Day 9	MD	11	8	Heart-CNS
		Rat	SZ	Day 0	MD	13	15	Heart-CNS
		Rat	SZ	Day 0	MD	20	72	Omphalocele, skeletal
Brownscheidle and Davies (29)	1981	BB rat			MDI	19–NB	23	Brain, eye, skeletal, placental cysts
Baker et al (30)	1981	Rat	SZ	Day 6	MD	20	17	Lumbosacral
		Rat	SZ	Day 12	MD	20	0	Lumbosacral
		Rat	SZ	Day 6	MDI	20	5	Lumbosacral
Eriksson et al (31)	1982	Rat	SZ	Before pregnancy	MD	18–22	17–23	Skeletal
		Rat	SZ	Before pregnancy	MDI	18–22	0–3	Skeletal
Brownscheidle et al (32)	1983	BB rat			MDI	NB	20–37	CNS, skeletal, eye
		BB rat			MDI$_{pump}$	NB	10	CNS, skeletal, eye
Eriksson et al (33)	1983	Rat	SZ	Before pregnancy	MD	20	19	Skeletal
		Rat	SZ	Before pregnancy	MDII	20	0–6	Skeletal
Funaki and Mikamo (34)	1983	Chinese hamster			MD	18	4	CNS, skeletal, tail, omphalocele

Reference	Year	Species		Treatment				Malformations
Eriksson (35)	1984	Rat	SZ	Before pregnancy	MD	18–22	14	Skeletal
		Rat	SZ	Before pregnancy	MDZ	20	16	Skeletal
Ornoy et al (36)	1984	Rat	SZ	Day 5	MD	20–21	—	Placental cysts
		Rat	SZ	Day 12	MD	20–21	—	Placental cysts
Goldman et al (92)	1985	Rat	SZ	Day 6	MD	20	29	Neural tube, skeletal
					MDAA	20	9	Neural tube, skeletal
Eriksson et al (85)	1985	BB rat			MDII	20	0–6	Skeletal, CNS
Eriksson et al (37)	1986	Rat (U)	SZ	Before pregnancy	MD/MDII	20	4–19	Skeletal
		Rat (H)	SZ	Before pregnancy	MD/MDII	20	0	
Zusman and Ornoy (89)	1986	Rat	SZ	Day 5	SD	9–17	0–18	CNS, yolk sac
		CD rat			SD	9–17	0–15	CNS, yolk sac
Eriksson et al (91)	1986	Rat (U)	SZ	Before pregnancy	MD	11/20	32/12	CNS, skeletal
					MDARI	11/20	32/13	CNS, skeletal
Eriksson and Eriksson (86)	1987	Rat (U)	SZ	Before pregnancy	MDII$_{pump}$	20	0–8	Skeletal
Eriksson (90)	1987	Rat (U)	SZ	Before pregnancy	MD	20	3–17	Skeletal
		Rat (H)	SZ	Before pregnancy	MD	20	0	
		Rat (U/H)	SZ	Before pregnancy	MD	20	5–19	Skeletal

MDI$_{pump}$ = MDI with osmotic insulin pump, MDZ = MD and zinc supplement, BB rat = spontaneously diabetic rat strain, rat (U) = Uppsala substrain of Sprague-Dawley rat, rat H = Hanover substrain of Sprague-Dawley rats, MDAA = MD and arachidonic acid supplement, MDII = MDI with interrupted insulin treatment during pregnancy, CD rat = Cohen diabetic rat (from an inbred glucose intolerant rat strain), MDARI = MD with aldose reducase inhibitor treatment, rat (U/H) = F$_1$ hybrid between U and H rats.
For further explanation of remaining abbreviations, see Table 1.1a.

TABLE 1.2. Congenital malformations (CM) in offspring of animals with elevated levels of different sugars.

Reference	Year	Animal	Sugar	Mode of administration	Type(s) of CM
Mandrey (38)	1940	Rat	Galactose	Diet supplement	Cataract
Bannon et al (39)	1945	Rat	Galactose	Diet supplement	Cataract
Segal and Bernstein (40)	1963	Rat	Galactose	Diet supplement	Cataract
Clavert et al (41)	1972	Rabbit	D-glucose	Amniotic sac instillation	Skeletal
Clavert and Wolff-Quenot (42)	1973	Rabbit	D-glucose	Amniotic sac instillation	Skeletal
Hughes et al (43)	1974	Chicken	Various	Injection into egg	Trunk, tail, CNS
Ornoy and Cohen (44)	1980	Glucose-intolerant rat	Sucrose	Diet supplement	CNS, heart
Buchanan et al (45)	1985	Rat	D-mannose	12 h IV infusion	CNS, heart, eye
		Rat	D-glucose	12 h IV infusion	
Zusman and Ornoy (89)	1986	SZ rat	Sucrose	Diet supplement	CNS, yolk sac
		CD rat	Sucrose	Diet supplement	CNS, yolk sac

IV = intravenous, SZ rat = streptozotocin-diabetic rat. For further explanation of remaining abbreviations, see Table 1.1b.

In two studies, Endo and collaborators examined the frequency of chromosomal aberrations in offspring of alloxan-diabetic mice made diabetic at least three days before conception (22,24). In the first study thin pieces of minced tissue from fetal limbs, tails, and palates were cultured for three to five days and prepared for chromosomal analysis. The frequency of cells with polyploidy, aneuploidy, chromosomal gaps and breaks was lowest in normal offspring, slightly higher in offspring of diabetic mice, and highest in malformed offspring of diabetic mice. In the second study chromosomal analysis was performed in blastocysts removed from the uteri of pregnant diabetic mice on gestational day 3. In addition to a marked decrease in the number of viable blastocysts, there was also an increased incidence of polyploidy, aneuploidy, and chromosomal breaks in these early embryos, confirming the findings of the first study but at a much earlier gestational age.

The first published study on fetal malformations in spontaneously diabetic animals confirmed several of the observations previously made in experimental diabetic pregnancies (29). Neonatal mortality and the frequency of gross malformations were increased in the offspring of diabetic BB rats, whereas no malformations were observed in BB rat fetuses when neither of the parents or only the father was diabetic, or in the offspring of control nondiabetic rats. In a recent study of the spontaneously diabetic Chinese hamster, Funaki and Mikano examined both early blastocyst-embryonic development as well as fetal outcome in diabetic pregnancy (34). They found no difference in the chromosomal aberration rate between embryos of diabetic hamsters and those of normal hamsters. Moreover, they did not observe any decrease in the number of ovulated ova, surviving embryos, or implantation sites in the diabetic hamsters compared with the normal ones. These results were not in accord with the data previously reported from studies in diabetic mice (22,24). However, an increase in the incidence of postimplantation deaths and fetal malformations in the offspring of the diabetic hamsters was noted. suggesting that the teratogenic influences appeared during embryogenesis, rather than at an early blastocyst stage. The conflicting results concerning preimplanted embryonic viability and cytogenetic characteristics may be strain-related. Funaki and Mikano suggested that experimentally diabetic mice may display a more irregular estrous cycle and consequently more chromosomal aberrations than the diabetic hamsters they used in their study.

Several investigators have reported that good metabolic control prevents fetal malformations. Baker and collaborators showed that in rats made diabetic with SZ on gestational day 6, insulin treatment from gestational days 6 through 13 decreased the occurrence of lumbosacral anomalies (30). When SZ was given on gestational day 12, no ossification anomalies were encountered in the offspring. Eriksson et al showed that offspring of rats with overt diabetes exhibited an increased incidence of two specific

TABLE 1.3. Congenital malformations (CM) in embryos cultured in vitro under diabetes-like conditions.

Reference	Year	Embryo	Culture start (d)	Culture duration (h)	Serum	Culture condition	Type of CM
Cockroft and Coppola (46)	1977	Rat	9.5	48	Rat	15 mg/mL D-glucose	Neural tube
Deuchar (47)	1979	Rat	10	24	Maternal rat	MD serum	Various
Sadler (48)	1980	Mouse	8.5	24	Rat	SD/MD serum	Neural tube
Sadler (49)	1980	Mouse	8.5	24	Rat	6–9 mg/mL D-glucose	Neural tube
Horton and Sadler (50)	1983	Mouse	8.5	24	Rat	8–32 mM β-hydroxybutyrate (β-HB)	Neural tube (mitochondriae)
Sadler and Horton (51)	1983	Mouse	8.5	24	Rat	MD/MDI serum	Neural tube
Garnham et al (52)	1983	Rat	9	48	Rat	10 mg/mL D-glucose	Neural tube
Lewis et al (53)	1983	Rat	9.5	48	Rat	6 mg/mL D-glucose $\pm$ 8mM β-HB	Neural tube brain, heart
Freinkel et al (54)	1984	Rat	9.5	48	Rat	1.5 mg/mL mannose	Neural tube
Cockroft (101)	1984	Rat	8.8–9.8	48–66	Rat	12–15 mg/mL D-glucose	Neural tube
Horton and Sadler (108)	1985	Mouse	8.5	24–48	Rat	8–32 mM β-HB	Neural tube mitochondriae

Reece et al (102)	1985	Rat	9.5	48	Rat	7.5 mg/mL D-glucose	Neural tube, neuroepithelial histology
Goldman et al (92)	1985	Mouse	8.3	48	Rat	8 mg/mL D-glucose ± arachidonic acid	Neural tube
Akazawa et al (98)	1986	Rat	9.5	48	Rat	Hypoglycemic serum	Neural tube
Ornoy et al (100)	1986	Rat	9.5	48	Rat	N/CD/SZ serum	Neural tube, yolk sac
		CD rat	9.5	48	Rat	N/CD/SZ serum	Neural tube, yolk sac
		SZ rat	9.5	48	Rat	N/CD/SZ serum	Neural tube, yolk sac
Pinter et al (103)	1986	Rat	9.5	48	Rat	7.5 mg/mL D-glucose	Neural tube, yolk sac
Pinter et al (106)	1986	Rat	9.5	48	Rat	9.5 mg/mL D-glucose ± arachidonic acid	Neural tube, yolk sac
Sadler et al (110)	1986	Mouse	8.5	24	Rat	SMI serum	Neural tube
Freinkel et al (113)	1986	Rat	9.5	48	Rat	SMI serum	Neural tube
Hod et al (105)	1986	Rat	9.5	48	Rat	3–12 mg/mL D-glucose ± ARI	Various
Brolin et al (104)	1986	Rat	9.5	48	Rat	12 mg/mL D-glucose ± ARI	Neural tube
Sadler and Hunter (99)	1987	Mouse	8.5	28	Rat	Hypoglycemic serum	Various
Hunter et al (109)	1987	Mouse	8.5	24	Rat	16–32 mM β-HB ± ribose	Various
Eriksson (90)	1987	Rat	9.5	48	Rat	6 mg/mL D-glucose ± 8mM β-HB	Various

SMI serum = somatomedin inhibitor-containing serum, ARI = aldose reductase inhibitor.
For explanation of remaining abbreviations, see Tables 1.1a, 1.1b, and 1.2.

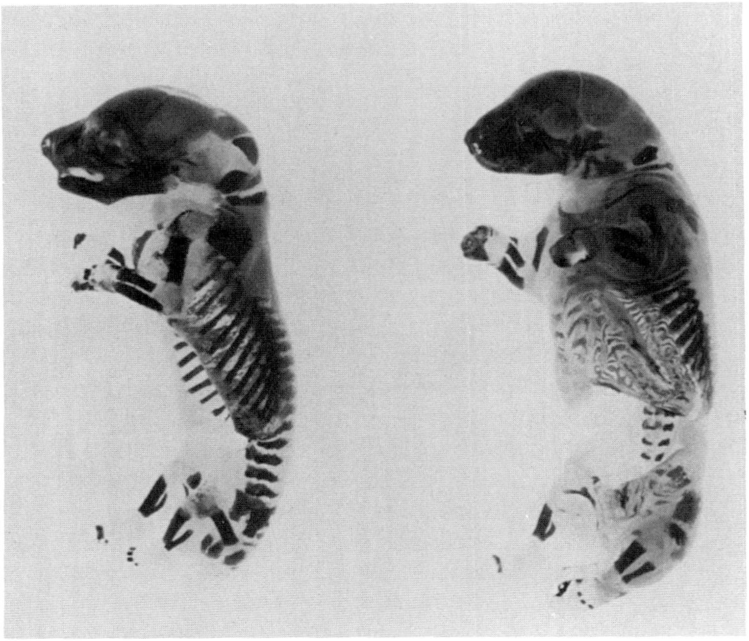

FIGURE 1.1. Two rat fetuses from a nondiabetic (left) and manifest diabetic (right) mother on gestational day 20. The skeleton is made visible by alizarin red staining. The fetus to the right shows micrognathia and a malformed left eye. (With kind permission of Teviot-Kimpton Publications.)

skeletal malformations, micrognathia (Figure 1.1) and caudal dysgenesis (Figure 1.2). Treatment of the mothers with insulin decreased the incidence of these malformations (31). In the diabetic BB rat, the incidence of malformations observed among animals treated with continuous insulin infusion via implanted osmotic minipumps was markedly lower than that among animals receiving insulin injections (protamine zinc or lente insulin) (32). In an attempt to define the teratogenic period and its relation to insulin effects, Eriksson et al subjected manifestly diabetic rats to a regimen of intermittent insulin treatment (33). Withdrawal of insulin in the diabetic rats during gestational days 2 through 8 resulted in both micrognathia (Figure 1.1) and caudal dysgenesis (Figure 1.2) in the offspring. This finding of an early teratogenic period with respect to skeletal malformations contrasted with the results of Baker et al, who suggested that the sensitive period of induction of lumbosacral anomalies in the rat was between gestational days 6 and 12. On the other hand, Ornoy and collaborators failed to produce malformations of the fetal skeleton by injecting high doses of SZ in normal pregnant rats on gestational day 5 or 12 (36).

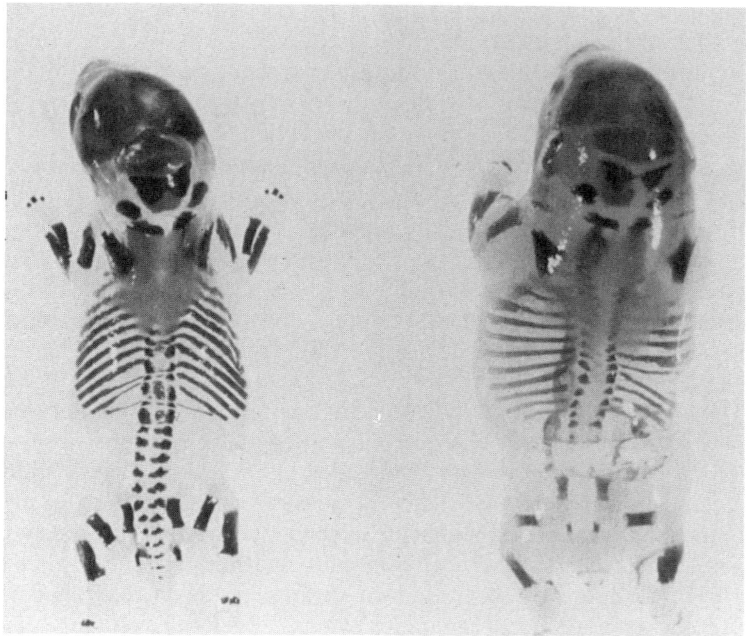

FIGURE 1.2. Two rat fetuses from a nondiabetic (left) and manifest diabetic (right) mother on gestational day 20, stained with alizarin red. The fetus of the diabetic mother shows lack of tail and no ossification in the caudal region, i.e., caudal (sacral) dysgenesis. (With kind permission of Teviot-Kimpton Publications.)

However, differences in the experimental protocols and in the types of anomalies and malformations studied, as well as in the rat strains used, may account for differences in the results. This view is further strengthened by the findings of two recent studies of the effects on fetal development of interrupted insulin treatment in BB rats (85) and malformation-prone SZ-diabetic rats (86). The BB rats were kept on a twice daily insulin treatment scheme except for a two day interruption and all fetal malformations occurred in the day 6–8 (3%) and day 8–10 (6%) interruption groups (85). In the SZ-diabetic rats, osmotic insulin pumps were placed in the animals to precisely control the maternal diabetic state except for two or four days during pregnancy (when the animals had no pumps at all). The malformations occurred in the day 6–8 (2%), day 8–10 (3%), day 6–10 (8%) and day 8–12 (2%) interruption groups (86). The combined findings in all these studies implicate pregnancy days 6–10 in the rat (roughly corresponding to weeks 2–4 in human gestation) as a period of maximal teratological susceptibility.

The importance of a genetic predisposition for the induction of congenital malformations has been suggested by a number of studies. When offspring of two related Sprague-Dawley rat substrains (U and H) were compared, striking differences in the malformation rate were detected, although the maternal diabetic state was of similar severity (37). Several other rat strains have been investigated, using similar preconceptual SZ-induction of diabetes, with no malformations detected, although the resorption rates were elevated (87,88). When the maldeveloped offspring (i.e., combined rates of malformations, resorptions and conceptuses with signs of delayed development) of glucose-intolerant Cohen rats and SZ-diabetic rats were compared on gestational days 9–17 they showed different patterns. The SZ-diabetic rats had more maldeveloped embryos on gestational day 9 (25 vs. 8%), day 11 (25 vs. 15%) and day 13 (13 vs. 0%), whereas the opposite was true on gestational day 15 (7 vs. 25%) and day 17 (11 vs. 25%) (89). It is therefore conceivable that genetic variations may explain the widely different incidences of congenital malformations observed in the offspring of diabetic animals. This question has been further addressed in a recent study where two different strains of rats with different malformation rates in diabetic pregnancy were compared (90). By cross-mating malformation-prone (U rats) with nonmalformation-prone (H) rats and using an F1-hybrid (G rats) of these two strains, it was possible to compare the outcome of diabetic pregnancies where genetically similar offspring were subjected to genetically different diabetic uterine environments, and to evaluate the effect of similar maternal diabetic environment on embryos with different genetic makeup. This study showed, as expected, that the maternal genome is of prime importance for the induction of congenital malformations (and fetal resorptions), but also, that the *fetal* genome is of great importance for the induction process (90).

Diabetic complications have been associated with increased sorbitol levels in the affected tissues. Embryos and fetuses of manifestly diabetic rats have also been shown to exhibit elevated levels of sorbitol (91). This increase was completely normalized in embryos, and partly normalized in fetal livers and placentae, when the diabetic rat mother was treated with an aldose reductase inhibitor during pregnancy. There were, however, no differences between sorbitol levels in nonmalformed and malformed offspring, and the aldose reductase inhibitor treatment did not decrease the rate of malformations among embryos and fetuses of the diabetic rats (91). From this experimental study, it therefore appears that sorbitol accumulation may not be directly involved in the induction of congenital malformations in diabetic pregnancy.

Arachidonic acid disturbances, on the other hand, may be involved in the etiology of malformations produced by diabetic pregnancy as a study by Goldman and collaborators has suggested (92). These authors injected arachidonic acid to pregnant diabetic rats and found that the rate of skeletal defects in the offspring was reduced.

Additionally, a possible relationship between malformation rates and alterations in trace metal concentrations has been suggested. The total body concentration of zinc was decreased in fetuses of rats made diabetic with SZ 2 to 6 weeks before pregnancy (35). Fetal zinc deficiency and an increase in the rate of skeletal malformations in the offspring of the diabetic group persisted despite maternal zinc treatment during pregnancy. Copper concentrations were similar in the fetuses of normal and diabetic mothers, whereas fetal manganese concentration was increased in the offspring of diabetic rats, indicating that the observed fetal zinc deficiency did not simply reflect a general trace metal shortage. These results were substantiated by the recent demonstration of skeletal malformations in the offspring of nondiabetic U rats fed a zinc-deficient diet (55) and by Uriu-Hare and collaborators who reported similar trace metal findings in the offspring of two strains of rats made SZ-diabetic before pregnancy (87). Diabetes seems to induce a transport deficiency of zinc in late gestation (Eriksson & Thomas, in preparation) and early pregnancy (93) of the rat. Although further studies on fetal-embryologic trace metal handling are required, it appears that changes in trace metal levels in the embryo may have a teratogenic impact in diabetic pregnancy.

Mohr et al first reported the presence of excessive fibrin deposits in the placentas of alloxan-diabetic rats (17). Subsequently, several investigators have described histopathologic changes in the placentas of SZ-diabetic rats. The most severe of these alterations consisted of large cystic dilatations in the spongiosa layer of the placentas (25–27,36). Both in the cysts and in the spaces between the trophoblastic cells, there was an increased amount of mucopolysaccharide material. Such cystic vacuoles also have been demonstrated in diabetic BB rats (spontaneously diabetic rat strain) (29). In SZ-diabetic rats, an increased placental weight (25,31,56) and increased glycogen (27,36,56) and lipid (36,56) contents have been repeatedly demonstrated. The functional importance of these changes in placental morphology is difficult to assess. However, a number of recent studies report compromised placental function in diabetic pregnancy (57,58,94,95,96,112). The blood flow in the placenta of manifestly diabetic rats was reduced (58,112) and the accumulation of radioactive alpha-aminoisobutyric acid in the fetuses of mildly diabetic guinea pigs and diabetic rats was found to be decreased (57,94). Disturbances in the handling of glucose and amino acids have also been demonstrated in diabetic rat pregnancy (95,96,112). The net flux of glucose and neutral amino acids from mother to fetus was found to be increased in manifestly diabetic rat pregnancy compared to normal pregnancy (95,112). When the glucose transfer in late gestation was studied in an experimental situation where both the maternal and fetal side of the placenta were catheterized simultaneously, it was found that for a given maternal-fetal glucose gradient the placenta of the diabetic rats was less able to transfer glucose than normal placenta.

This was due to a large back-flux of glucose from fetus to mother, which was present despite a huge concentration gradient between the two circulatory systems in the diabetic rat (96).

Increased Levels of Different Sugars In vivo

It has been reported that fetal malformations occur in several animal models after in vivo administration of different sugars (Table 1.2). In these studies, elevated embryo-fetal sugar levels correlated with increased rates of fetal malformations. Several early studies showed that feeding a diet rich in galactose to rats during gestation led to the development of cataracts in the offspring (38–40). In a more recent study, a diet high in sucrose resulted in increased resorption rates in normal rats and further increased an already elevated resorption frequency in a strain of rats with reduced glucose tolerance (44). Surprisingly, however, the rate of fetal malformations increased with sucrose feeding in normal rats, but no further increase above the basic malformation rate occurred in the inbred strain. In a more recent study, the occurrence of maldevelopment (rate of malformations, resorptions and conceptuses with signs of delayed development) in the offspring of control, SZ-diabetic, and Cohen glucose-intolerant rats increased when these groups were fed a sucrose diet with the embryos/fetuses evaluated on gestational days 9, 11, 13, 15, or 17 (89).

Clavert and collaborators infused glucose directly into the amniotic sac of rabbits on gestational day 14 and examined the effects on day 20 (41,42). They found increased fetal mortality and an increased malformation rate among the surviving offspring. On the other hand, injection of cortisone into the amniotic sacs resulted in a number of fetuses with cleft palate, but not in the type of malformations that had been induced with glucose. Malformation rates after combined treatment with glucose and cortisone were similar to those with either agent alone. The teratogenic effects of glucose were found to be specific for the D form and largely independent of the osmolarity of the injected solution. A number of sugars, D-glucose, L-glucose, D-mannose, fructose, sucrose, maltose, lactose, trehalose, and raffinose) induce trunk, tail, and central nervous system (CNS) malformations in chickens when injected into the egg after the start of incubation (43). Considered together, these studies suggest that embryonic exposure to high concentrations of glucose may be of particular teratologic interest, since increased rates of skeletal and other malformations result when glucose is instilled into the amniotic sac, injected into the egg, or added to the maternal diet as a component of sucrose.

Minor transient elevations in maternal glucose levels do not appear to hamper embryonic development. For example, Buchanan and collaborators infused D-glucose for 12 hours into pregnant nondiabetic rats on gestational days 9.5 through 10.0 to achieve transient elevation of plasma glucose levels and detected no abnormalities in the offspring on gestational day 11.5 (45). In contrast, infusion of D-mannose (plasma levels around 10 mM; glucose 3 to 5 mM) for the same period resulted in dysmorphic changes in 99% of the offspring. The teratogenicity of D-mannose has also been studied in vitro (54). The same authors have also studied the effects of short periods of hypoglycemia in vivo and found a slightly increased malformation rate and signs of retarded development (97).

In vitro Studies

In vitro investigations of diabetic pregnancy have been performed mainly in the whole-embryo culture system developed by New (59), using rodent embryos. Two principal conditions have been employed to study embryologic growth and development: incubation in serum from diabetic animals, and in media containing excess glucose and/or β-hydroxybutyrate (Table 1.3). Deuchar was the first to examine the in vitro effects of diabetic serum, using day-10 rat embryos cultured for 24 hours in watch-glasses (47). The diabetic state was induced by SZ injection on the day after mating, and serum for the cultures was obtained by heart puncture of the mothers at the time of explantation. Embryos from normal rats showed better development, regardless of the source of serum in which they were cultured. Sadler and collaborators also examined the effects of whole diabetic serum on embryologic growth and development (48,51). In one study they cultured day-8 mouse embryos for 24 hours in serum obtained from normal, mildly diabetic, and severely diabetic male rats and found that younger embryos had a higher rate of neural closure defects than older ones. They also examined the effect of insulin treatment of the diabetic serum donors (rats). Insulin therapy had a beneficial effect on day-8 mouse embryos, since the resulting normoglycemic and hyperglycemic sera produced malformation rates intermediate to those observed in cultures with either control serum or with serum from untreated diabetic rats. The addition of insulin directly to serum collected from untreated diabetic rats failed to reduce the rate of abnormalities,and the addition of insulin, even at high concentration, to normal rat serum did not produce malformations. On the other hand, serum from rats with hypoglycemia (<1 mg/mL) due to insulin therapy did produce malformations at a rate that was reduced when glucose concentration in the culture medium was normalized. Similar findings have been reported in other studies where embryos have been subjected to serum from rats with low glucose levels (98,99). In a large study the effects of several different sera on embryonic development in vitro were compared. The result showed that diabetic serum yielded malformations *also* when the diabetic serum donors had been given an insulin injection in order to normalize glucose levels (100).

Cockroft and Coppola reported that the addition of 15 mg/mL of D-glucose induced severe malformations and growth retardation in 48-hour culture day-9 rat embryos. When corrected for osmolarity changes due to elevated glucose levels, the frequency of severe malformations decreased (46). This frequency also declined when less D-glucose was added, or when L-glucose was used instead of D-glucose. Other investigators have studied the effects of elevated glucose levels in otherwise normal serum in embryo culture systems. In day-8 mouse embryos cultured for 24 hours, Sadler (49) demonstrated both dose- and age-dependent effects of the glucose addition. He found that younger embryos more frequently exhibited neural tube closure defects than did older ones. In addition, more embryos were affected at the higher than at the lower glucose concentrations. Garnham et al (52) investigated the time scale of glucose-induced teratogenesis by exposing day-9 rat embryos to a glucose concentration of 10 mg/mL for different time periods during a 48-hour culture period. The initial 21 hours of culture constituted the teratologically most susceptible period, during which 42% of the embryos developed "squirrel-like" neural tube fusion defects in comparison with, for example, the subsequent 27 hours of culture during which only an 11% rate of "squirrel-like" embryos was found. Similar results indicating that younger embryos are more susceptible than older ones have been reported by Cockroft. His study suggests that the time period between gestational days 9.5–10.0 may be the in vitro stage of highest teratological sensitivity towards D-glucose (101). A number of other in vitro investigations indicate that one of the primary effects of a hyperglycemic environment is an alteration of the development of the embryonic yolk sac (100,102,103).

Another effect of increased glucose levels, i.e., accumulation of sorbitol in embryos and membranes, has also been investigated in vitro and not found to be directly associated with embryonic malformation rate (104,105), as studies in vivo have suggested (91). On the other hand, the findings of a beneficial effect of arachidonic acid supplementation to diabetic rats in vivo (92) have been corroborated by the addition of this compound to embryo cultures with elevated glucose levels, resulting in a decrease in embryonic maldevelopment (92,106).

In vitro studies of another potentially teratogenic factor in diabetic pregnancy, hyperketonemia, have also been performed. Horton and Sadler (50) found neural tube closure defects in day-8 mouse embryos cultured for 24 hours in the presence of 8 to 32 mmol/L of β-hydroxybutyrate. Younger embryos were more frequently affected than older ones. Higher concentrations of the compound also led to higher rates of malformations. Furthermore, electron microscopic examination of the affected neuroepithelial cells, and of the surrounding mesenchyme and ectoderm, revealed numerous grossly swollen and morphologically distorted mitochondria, showing loss of matrix density and only a few identifiable cristae, and thereby strongly suggesting disturbed function. This group has examined the effects of increased levels of ketone bodies in great morphological and biochemical detail (107,108) and noted that hyperketonemia leads to decreased activity in the embryonic hexose monophosphate shunt (109). These observations are of interest in view of the finding by Lewis et al of a synergistic action between (sub)teratogenic doses of 6 mg/mL D-glucose and 8 mmol/L β-hydroxybutyrate in day-9 rat embryos cultured for 48 hours (53). Malformations occurred at a higher rate following the combined treatment than after addition of the individual compounds. In another recent study, embryos from two different rat strains (U and H) were subjected to identical teratological concentrations of glucose and/or β-hydroxybutyrate in vitro with no apparent difference in the outcome. This finding would suggest that the etiology of the malformations seen in vitro and in vivo may be different (90).

A recent study compared the teratogenicity of D-glucose and D-mannose and proposed the existence of a coupling between mannose-induced teratogenesis and the interruption of a glycolysis (54). In day-9 rat embryos cultured for 48 hours, both the high rate of mannose-related embryologic malformations and the impaired glycolytic flux (decreased lactic acid production) could be concomitantly overcome by the addition of excess glucose to the mannose-containing medium. Furthermore, the mannose-related teratogenic effects occurred mainly during the first 24 hours of culture, and an increase in the level of atmospheric oxygen during that period also decreased the rate of both neural and extraneural lesions (54). A different approach has been made in two recent investigations where the authors cultured mouse and rat embryos in serum from rats with increased levels of somatomedin inhibitors (110) and found this in vitro culture teratogenic in a dose-dependent manner (111,113).

Etiologic Reflections

Genetic Predisposition and Severity of Maternal Diabetic State

The two possible types of teratogenic influence on the growing embryo are genetic (hereditary) and environmental (diabetic intrauterine milieu). Animal models have provided evidence in favor of both elements in diabetic teratogenesis. The number of studies in which congenital malformations have been reported constitute only a small fraction of all the animal studies of diabetic pregnancy performed. Furthermore, the malformations and anomalies show great variations between different animals and experimental protocols. This suggests that susceptibility to the teratogen(s) of diabetic pregnancy is low and varies between different species. In the rat, there are striking differences in rates of teratogenesis even between apparently related strains (37,60). Some recent clinical reports link facial malformations to sacrocaudal malformations in human diabetic pregnancy (61,62). A rat model, which expresses similar skeletal aberrations—micrognathia and sacral dysgenesis—may therefore be a useful tool in studies of the etiologic relationships between disturbed maternal metabolism and skeletal malformations in the offspring. Another possible indication of genetic involvement is the finding of an increased rate of chromosomal aberrations in the malformed offspring of diabetic mice (22,24). The weight of evidence would favor the notion that the occurrence of malformations is linked to hereditary factors in diabetic pregnant animals. On the other hand, there are striking differences in the rates of malformations between diabetic and nondiabetic animals (of genetically susceptible strains), indicating that the diabetic environment plays an important role. Several studies have shown that tight metabolic control lowers the rate of both fetal malformations and perinatal mortality (20,29,31,32,33,37,85,86), but also that the genetic constitution of the offspring is important for embryonic maldevelopment in diabetic pregnancy (90). These findings suggest that the mechanism of diabetic teratogenesis may reside in an interplay between a genetically predisposed embryonic organism and an altered maternal environment at a specific time period during or before organogenesis. If this hypothesis is true, the teratogenic influence could involve a change in the transport of a certain factor or class of factors from mother to embryo. The net result might be an overaccumulation or underaccumulation of such factors in the embryo/fetus. Teratogenesis might therefore be considered in terms of either a *toxic* (overaccumulation in the conceptus) or a *starvation*-like (underaccumulation) effect.

Insulin Hypoglycemia

It is unlikely that fetal insulin acts as a teratogen, since the pancreatic β-cells producing this peptide are not present in the embryo during the major part of organogenesis, i.e., at the time when the malformations are likely to be induced. Furthermore, maternal insulin does not penetrate the late (63) or early (64) chorioallantoic placenta and, in analogy, it would not be expected to cross the preplacental membranes either. Even if significant quantities of maternal insulin were to cross the animal or human preplacenta, the teratologic role of insulin would still be dubious, since the diabetic pregnant mother suffers from hypoinsulinemia rather than hyperinsulinemia. In view of these considerations, the malformations observed in the offspring of rabbits, mice, and rats after administration of excessive doses of insulin to the mother have most probably been due to effects secondary to the insulin administration, i.e., hypoglycemia (65–72). This notion is strengthened by the finding that excessive amounts of insulin have failed to produce embryologic malformations in vitro (51) and that administration of insulin to diabetic animals decreases rather than increases the malformation rate. It is conceivable that the effect of a hypoglycemic state on fetal development results from a disturbance of substrate metabolism, possibly leading to impairment of energy-dependent cell functions, i.e., a starvation-like situation. The reports on hypoglycemia producing fetal retardation and malformations both in vivo (97) and in vitro (98,99) give further support to this hypothesis.

D-Glucose and Other Sugars

Experimental maternal diabetes with accompanying hyperglycemia induces fetal malformations, but malformations following the administration of hexoses to nondiabetic animals are rare. In vivo exposure of embryos to high levels of carbohydrates has resulted in various malformations in rodents and chickens (Table 1.2). Despite the disparity in the pattern of malformations in these reports, the hyperglycemic state was related to an increase in the rate of malformations. Further, in vitro studies have demonstrated disturbed embryologic development and malformation after addition of glucose to normal serum, and these effects have appeared to be both age- and dose-related (46,49,52). Hyperglycemia per se may therefore play a role in the teratogenesis of diabetic pregnancy. It is also apparent that increased intracellular sorbitol levels may not be directly involved in the etiology of the skeletal malformations encountered in vivo (91) or the neural tube closure defects seen in vitro (104,105). The "toxic" action of hyperglycemia may depend on other metabolic or genetic factors for the induction of major teratogenic effects. The possible modes of action of hyperglycemia are multiple, ranging from decreased hexose monophosphate shunt activity due to reduced uptake of ascorbic acid (73), to increased nonenzymatic glycosylation of embryo proteins, leading to altered function (74,75). The explanation proposed for mannose teratogenicity (45,54)—depression of the glycolytic pathway—may represent another "starvation" mechanism involving disturbed handling of carbohydrates in the embryo. The effects of supplementation of arachidonic acid to embryos cultured in elevated glucose levels, e.g., decreasing glucose-induced malformations and growth retardation, demand further investigations (92,106). If increased extracellular glucose levels cause arachidonic acid depletion in culture, in a manner analogous to the effect of corticosterone on susceptible embryonic palate cells, then disruption of either prostaglandin biosynthesis or membrane lipid composition (or both) are conceivable.

Ketone Bodies

Since changes in maternal lipid metabolism in diabetes often parallel the disturbances in glucose homeostasis, the arguments in favor of hyperglycemia as a teratogenic factor also could apply to hyperketonemia. The in vitro demonstration of morphologically distorted mitochondria in β-hydroxybutyrate-treated embryos (50) suggests disturbed energy metabolism in these embryos. However, the augmented teratogenic effect of β-hydroxybutyrate when added together with glucose in vitro (53) suggests a synergism between these compounds, which may occur also in diabetic pregnancy. The "toxic" influence of increased levels of ketone bodies could be mediated through a change in the fetal metabolism of glucose, possibly leading to an inhibition of energy metabolism (76). On the other hand, it has also been demonstrated that β-hydroxybutyrate inhibits pyrimidine (77) and purine (78) biosynthesis in fetal rat brain. Furthermore, Hunter and co-workers have recently reported decreased hexose monophosphate shunt activity in embryos cultured in the presence of elevated β-hydroxybutyrate levels. This finding suggests a link between increased ketone body levels and decreased RNA/DNA biosynthesis due to lack of pentose precursors (109).

Trace Metals

Recent investigations suggest a relation between diabetic teratogenesis and trace metal disorders. Manifestly diabetic rats displayed disturbances of both maternal and fetal trace metal levels, in particular a reduced fetal zinc concentration, which was refractory to zinc treatment of the mother (35,87). These ideas are strengthened by the findings of decreased transport of zinc in late and early diabetic rat gestation (93). When nondiabetic rats of this malformation-prone substrain were fed a specially prepared diet poor in zinc, the fetuses exhibited similar degrees of zinc deficiency. In addition, these fetuses also showed skeletal malformations of a type closely resembling those seen in offspring of diabetic rats (55). These findings are interesting since zinc deficiency may be involved in teratologic processes both in humans (79,80) and in animals (81). Mechanisms likely to decrease embryo-fetal uptake of zinc in diabetic pregnancy have not been described, but an established zinc deficiency could have several possible teratogenic actions. For example, this trace metal serves as a cofactor for a number of enzymes, such as thymidine kinase, DNA-polymerase, and superoxide dismutase, and a deficiency might therefore inhibit the biosynthesis of DNA or affect the defense against free oxygen radicals in the conceptus (82–84).

Other Agents

The demonstration that serum fractions containing somatomedin inhibitory activity are teratogenic to embryos in vitro, is intriguing and should be evaluated further (111,113). Until the chemical nature of the inhibitor(s) is clarified, it is, however, difficult to assess the full importance of somatomedin inhibitors for the teratogenicity of diabetic pregnancy.

Conclusions

The precise nature of the teratogenic principle (or principles) operating in diabetic pregnancy remains unclear. Comparison of malformation rates between different substrains of Sprague-Dawley rats has shown marked differences in the occurrence of diabetes-induced malformations. These findings suggest that congenital malformations in diabetic pregnancy may result from a teratogenic insult in genetically predisposed individuals. Malformations in fetuses of diabetic animals seem to arise from teratogenic insult(s) early in pregnancy corresponding to gestational weeks 2–4 in human gestation. Hyperglycemia and hyperketonemia may be of teratologic significance singly, or in combination. Insulin itself does not appear to be directly teratogenic, whereas prolonged periods of extreme hypoglycemia may be harmful to the growing embryo. The glucose-induced disturbances in embryonic development may be partly normalized by arachidonic acid supplement, and mimicked by subjecting embryos to somatomedin inhibitory activity. Disturbed levels of trace metals, primarily zinc, may also be a significant factor in the production of congenital malformations. The increased rate of malformations in diabetic pregnancy, therefore, appears to be multifactorial in origin.

Acknowledgments. The work by the author referred to in this review was supported by the Swedish Medical Research Council (grant nos. 12X-07475, 12X-109, 12P-6346), the Bank of Sweden Tercentenary Foundation, the 'Expressen' Prenatal Research Foundation, the Family Ernfors Fund, the Nordic Insulin Fund, the Novo Industri A/S, the Swedish Diabetes Association, the Swedish Society of Medical Sciences, the University of Uppsala, and the Juvenile Diabetes Foundation (grant no. 185 544).

References

1. Duncan JM (1982) On puerperal diabetes. Trans Obstet Soc London 24:256–85.
2. Mølsted-Pedersen L, Tygstrup I, Pedersen J (1964) Congenital malformations in newborn infants of diabetic women. Correlation with maternal diabetic vascular complications. Lancet 1:1124–6.
3. Pedersen J (1977) The pregnant diabetic and her newborn ed 2. Copenhagen, Munksgaard, pp 1–280.
4. Freinkel N (1982) Of pregnancy and progeny. Banting Lecture. Diabetes 29:1023–35.
5. Mills JL (1982) Malformations in infants of diabetic mothers. Teratology 25:385–94.
6. Kucera J (1971) Rate and type of congenital anomalies among offspring of diabetic women. J Reprod Med 7:61–70.
7. Pedersen JF, Mølsted-Pedersen L (1982) Early growth delay predisposes the fetus in diabetic pregnancy to congenital malformation. Lancet 1:737.

8. Eriksson UJ, Lewis NJ, Freinkel N (1984) Growth retardation during early organogenesis in embryos of experimentally diabetic rats. Diabetes 33:281–4.
9. Spiers PS (1982) Does growth retardation predispose the fetus to congenital malformation? Lancet 1:312–4.
10. Tchobroutsky C, Breart GL, Rambaud DC, Henrion R (1985) Correlation between fetal defects and early growth delay observed by ultrasound. Lancet 1:706–7.
11. Ross OA, Spector S (1952) Production of congenital abnormalities in mice by alloxan. Am J Dis Child 84:647–8.
12. Bartelheimer H, Kloos K (1952) Die Auswirkung des experimentellen Diabetes auf Gravidität und Nachkommenschaft. Z Gesamte Exp Med 119:246–65.
13. Kreshover SJ, Clough W, Bear DM (1953) Prenatal influences on tooth development. I. Alloxan diabetes in rats. J Dent Res 32:246–61.
14. Fujimoto S, Sumi T, Kuzukawa S, Tonoike H, Miyoshi T, Nakamura S (1958) The genesis of experimental anomalies—fetal anomalies in reference to experimental diabetes in rabbit. J Osaka City Med Ctr 7:62–66 (in Japanese).
15. Koskenoja M (1961) Alloxan diabetes in the pregnant mouse. Acta Ophthalmol [Suppl] (Copenh) 68:1–92.
16. Watanabe G, Ingalls TH (1963) Congenital malformation in the offspring of alloxan-diabetic mice. Diabetes 12:66–72.
17. Mohr U, Althoff J, Wrba H (1964) Morphologische Veränderungen der Rattenplazenta beim Alloxandiabetes. Naturwissenschaften 51:440.
18. Barashnev YI (1965) Malformation of fetal brain resulting from alloxan diabetes in mother. Fed Proc 24:382–86.
19. Endo A (1966) Teratogenesis in diabetic mice treated with alloxan prior to conception. Arch Environ Health 12:492–500.
20. Horii K, Watanabe G, Ingalls TH (1966) Experimental diabetes in pregnant mice: prevention of congenital malformations in offspring by insulin. Diabetes 15:194–204.
21. Takano K, Nishimura H (1967) Congenital malformations induced by alloxan diabetes in mice and rats. Anat Rec 158:303–12.
22. Endo A, Ingalls TH (1968) Chromosomal anomalies in embryos of diabetic mice. Arch Environ Health 16:316–25.
23. Ichikari I (1970) Experimental studies concerning the prevention of diabetic embryopathy. Prevention of congenital malformations in alloxan-diabetic pregnant mice by the oral application of tolbutamide. Congenital Anomalies 10:29–40 (in Japanese).
24. Yamamoto M, Endo A, Watanabe G, Ingalls TH (1971) Chromosomal aneuploidies and polyploidies in embryos of diabetic mice. Arch Environ Health 22:468–75.
25. Prager R, Abramovici A, Liban E, Laron Z (1974) Histopathological changes in the placenta of streptozotocin induced diabetic rats. Diabetologia 10:89–91.
26. Emmrich P, Caffier P (1976) Plazentare Veränderungen bei Ratten mit Streptozotocin-diabetes. Endokrinologie 67:79–84.
27. Liban E, Abramovici A, Sporn J, Prager R, Laron Z (1976) Morphological and biochemical changes in the placenta of streptozotocin-induced diabetic rats. Harefuah 90:508–13 (in Hebrew, English abstract, pp 546–47).

28. Deuchar EM (1977) Embryonic malformations in rats, resulting from maternal diabetes: preliminary observations. J Embryol Exp Morphol 41:93–9.
29. Brownscheidle CM, Davies DL (1981) Diabetes in pregnancy: a preliminary study of the pancreas, placenta and malformations in the BB Wistar rat. Placenta 33 [Suppl]:203–16.
30. Baker L, Egler JM, Klein SM, Goldman AS (1981) Meticulous control of diabetes during organogenesis prevents congenital lumbosacral defects in rats. Diabetes 30:955–59.
31. Eriksson UJ, Dahlström E, Larsson KS, Hellerström C (1982) Increased incidence of congenital malformations in the offspring of diabetic rats and their prevention by maternal insulin therapy. Diabetes 31:1–6.
32. Brownscheidle CM, Wootten, V, Mathieu MH, Davis DL, Hofman IA (1983) The effects of maternal diabetes on fetal maturation and neonatal health. Metabolism 32 [Suppl]:148–55.
33. Eriksson UJ, Dahlström E, Hellerström C (1983) Diabetes in pregnancy: Skeletal malformations in the offspring of diabetic rats after intermittent withdrawal of insulin in early gestation. Diabetes 31:1141–45.
34. Funaki K, Mikano K (1983) Developmental-stage-dependent teratogenic effects of maternal spontaneous diabetes in the Chinese hamster. Diabetes 32:637–43.
35. Eriksson UJ (1984) Diabetes in pregnancy: Fetal growth retardation, congenital malformations and feto-maternal concentrations of zinc, copper and manganese in the rat. J Nutr 114:477–86.
36. Ornoy A, Merin B, Zusman I, Granat M, Barash V, Shafris E (1984) Placental and skeletal changes in fetuses of streptozotocin-diabetic rats. In: Shafrir E, Renold AE (eds) Lessons from Animal Diabetes. John Libbey & Co. Ltd, London, pp 775–81.
37. Eriksson UJ, Dahlström VE, Lithell HO (1986) Diabetes in pregnancy: influence of genetic background and maternal diabetic state on the incidence of skeletal malformations in the fetal rat. Acta Endocrinol (Copenh) 112(Suppl 277):66–73
38. Mandrey J (1940) Development of cataract in the embryonic lens of the albino rat. Anat Rec 76 [Suppl 2]:92.
39. Bannon SL, Higginbottom RM, McConnel JM, Kaan HW (1945) Development of galactose cataract in the albino rat embryo. Arch Ophthalmol 33:224–28.
40. Segal S, Bernstein H (1963) Observations on cataract formation in the newborn offspring of rats fed a high-galactose diet. J Pediatr 62:363–70.
41. Clavert A, Wolff-Quenot MJ, Buck P (1972) Etude de l'action embryopathique du glucose en injection intraamniotique. C R Soc Biol (Paris) 166:1789–92.
42. Clavert A, Wolff-Quenot MJ. (1973) Etude du mode d'action embryopathique du glucose en injection dans le liquide ovulaire du Lapin. C R Soc Biol (Paris) 167:1452–4.
43. Hughes AF, Freeman FB, Fadem T (1974) The teratogenic effects of sugars on the chick embryo. J Embryol Exp Morphol 32:661–74.
44. Ornoy A, Cohen AM (1980) Teratogenic effects of sucrose diet in diabetic and non-diabetic rats. Isr J Med Sci 16:789–91.
45. Buchanan TA, Freinkel N, Lewis NJ, et al (1985) Fuel-mediated teratogenesis.

Use of D-mannose to modify organogenesis in the rat embryo in vivo. J Clin Invest 75:1927–34.

46. Cockroft DL, Coppola PT (1977) Teratogenic effects of excess glucose on head-fold rat embryos in culture. Teratology 16:141–6.

47. Deuchar E (1979) Culture *in vitro* as a means of analysing the effect of maternal diabetes on embryonic development in rats. In: Elliott K, O'Connor M (eds) Pregnancy metabolism, diabetes and the fetus. CIBA Foundation Series 63, Excerpta Medica, Amsterdam, pp 181–97.

48. Sadler TW (1980) Effects of maternal diabetes on early embryogenesis. I. The teratogenic potential of diabetic serum. Teratology 21:339–47.

49. Sadler TW (1980) Effects of maternal diabetes on early embryogenesis. II. Hyperglycemia-induced exencephaly. Teratology 21:349–56.

50. Horton WE Jr, Sadler TW (1983) Effects of maternal diabetes on early embryogenesis. Alternations in morphogenesis produced by the ketone body, β-hydroxybutyrate. Diabetes 32:610–6.

51. Sadler TW, Horton WE Jr (1983) Effects of maternal diabetes on early embryogenesis: the role of insulin and insulin therapy. Diabetes 32:1070–4.

52. Garnham EA, Beck F, Clarke CA, Stanisstreet M (1983) Effects of glucose on rat embryos in culture. Diabetologia 25:291–95.

53. Lewis NJ, Akazawa S, Freinkel N (1983) Teratogenesis from β-Hydroxybutyrate during organogenesis in rat embryo organ culture and enhancement by subteratogenic glucose. Diabetes 32 [Suppl 1]:11A.

54. Freinkel N, Lewis NJ, Akazawa S, Roth SI, Gorman L (1984) The honeybee syndrome—implications of the teratogenicity of mannose in rat-embryo culture. N Engl J Med 310:223–30.

55. Styrud J, Dahlström VE, Eriksson UJ (1986) Induction of skeletal malformations in the offspring of rats fed a zinc-deficient diet. Uppsala J Med Sci 91:29–36.

56. Diamant YZ, Metzger BE, Freinkel N, Shafir E (1982) Placental lipid and glycogen content in human and experimental diabetes mellitus. Am J Obstet Gynecol 144:5–11.

57. Saintonge J, Coté R (1983) Intrauterine growth retardation and diabetic pregnancy: Two types of fetal malnutrition. Am J Obstet Gynecol 146:194–8.

58. Eriksson UJ, Jansson L (1984) Diabetes in pregnancy: Decreased placental blood flow and disturbed fetal development in the rat. Pediatr Res 18:735–8.

59. New DAT (1978) Whole-embryo culture and the study of mammalian embryos during organogenesis. Biol Rev 53:81–122.

60. Eriksson UJ, Dahlström VE, Styrud J (1985) Metabolically determined teratogenesis: malformations and maternal diabetes. Biochem Soc Trans 13:79–82.

61. Grix A Jr (1982) Invited editorial comment: malformations in infants of diabetic mothers. Am J Med Genet 13:131–7.

62. Johnson JP, Carey JC, Gooch WM III, Petersson J, Bettie JF (1983) Femoral hypoplasia-unusual facies syndrome in infants of diabetic mothers. J Pediatr 102:866–72.

63. Goodner CM, Freinkel N (1961) Carbohydrate metabolism in pregnancy. IV. Studies on the permeability of the rat placenta to I^{131} insulin. Diabetes 10:383–92.

64. Widness JA, Goldman AS, Susa JB, Oh W, Schwartz R (1983) Impermeability of the rat placenta to insulin during organogenesis. Teratology 28:327–32.
65. Chomette G (1955) Entwicklungsstörnungen nach Insulinschock beim trächtigen Kaninchen. Beitr Pathol Anat 115:439–51.
66. Brinsmade A, Büchner F, Rübsaamen H (1956) Missbildungen am Kaninchenembryo durch Insulininjektion beim Mettertier. Naturwissenschaften 43:259.
67. Brinsmade AB (1957) Entwicklungsstörnungen am Kaninchenembryo nach Glukosemangel beim trächtigen Muttertier. Beitr Pathol Anat 117:140–53.
68. Lichtenstein H, Guest GM, Warkany J (1951) Abnormalities of offspring of white rats given protamin zinc insulin during pregnancy. Proc Soc Exp Biol Med 78:398–402.
69. Smithberg M, Runner MN (1963) Teratogenic effects of hypoglycemic treatments in inbred strains of mice. Am J Anat 113:479–89.
70. Love EJ, Kinch RAH, Stevenson JAF (1964) The effect of protamine zinc insulin on the outcome of pregnancy in the normal rat. Diabetes 13:44–8.
71. Hannah RS, Moore KL (1971) Effects of fasting and insulin on skeletal development in rats. Teratology 4:135–40.
72. Ream JR Jr, Weingarten PL, Pappas AM (1970) Evaluation of the prenatal effects of massive doses of insulin in rats. Teratology 3:29–32.
73. Ely JTA. (1981) Hyperglycemia and major congenital anomalies. N Engl J Med 305:833.
74. Miller E, Hare JW, Cloherty JP, Dunn PJ, Gleason RE, Soeldner S, Kitzmiller JL (1981) Elevated hemoglobin A_{1c} in early pregnancy and major congenital anomalies in infants of diabetic mothers. N Engl J Med 304:1331–4
75. Kennedy L, Baynes JW (1984) Non-enzymatic glycosylation and the chronic complications of diabetes: an overview. Diabetologia 26:93–8.
76. Magee BA, Potezny N, Rofe AM, Conyers AJ (1979) The inhibition of malignant cell growth by ketone bodies. Aust J Exp Biol Med Sci 57:529–39.
77. Bhasin S, Shambaugh III GE (1982) Fetal fuels. V. Ketone bodies inhibit pyrimidine biosynthesis in fetal rat brain. Am J Physiol 243:E234–9.
78. Shambaugh GE III, Angulo MC, Koehler RR (1984) Fetal fuels. VII. Ketone bodies inhibit synthesis of purines in fetal rat brain. Am J Physiol 247 (Endocrinol Metab 10): E111–7.
79. Hambidge KM, Neldner KH, Walravens PA (1975) Zinc, acrodermatitis enteropathica, and congenital malformations. Lancet 1:577–8.
80. Jameson S (1976) Effects of zinc deficiency in human reproduction. Thesis Acta Med Scand [Suppl 593]:1–89.
81. Hurley LS (1966) Swenerton H. Congenital malformations resulting from zinc deficiency in rats. Proc Soc Exp Biol Med 123:692–7.
82. Dreosti IE, Grey PC, Wilkins PJ (1972) Deoxyribonucleic acid synthesis, protein synthesis and teratogenesis in zinc-deficient rats. S Afr Med J 46:1585–8.
83. Prasad AS, Oberleas D (1974) Thymidine kinase activity and incorporation of thymidine into DNA in zinc-deficient tissue. J Lab Clin Med 83:634–9.
84. Duncan JR, Hurley LS (1978) Thymidine kinase and DNA polymerase activity in normal and zinc deficient developing rat embryos. Proc Soc Exp Biol Med 159:39–43.

85. Eriksson UJ, Baird JD, Turnbull DM, et al (1985) Timed interruption of insulin therapy in diabetic BB/E rat pregnancy: effects on fetal outcome. 12th Congr IDF, Madrid, Spain, September 23–28, 1985 (abstract).
86. Eriksson RSM, Eriksson UJ (1987) Diabetes in pregnancy: effects on fetal outcome by interrupted insulin treatment of the pregnant rat. Submitted for publication.
87. Uriu-Hare J, Stern JS, Reaven GM, et al (1985) The effect of maternal diabetes on trace element status and fetal development in the rat. Diabetes 34:1031–40.
88. Giavini E, Broccia ML, Prati M, et al (1986) Effects of streptozotocin-induced diabetes on fetal development in the rat. Teratology 34:81–8.
89. Zusman I, Ornoy A (1986) The effects of maternal diabetes and high sucrose diets on the intrauterine development of rat fetuses. Diab Res 3:153–9.
90. Eriksson UJ (1987) Importance of genetic predisposition and maternal environment for the occurrence of congenital malformations in offspring of diabetic rats. Accepted for publication.
91. Eriksson UJ, Naeser P, Brolin SE (1986) Increased accumulation of sorbitol in embryos of manifest diabetic rats. Diabetes 35:1356–63.
92. Goldman AS, Baker L, Piddington R, et al (1985) Hyperglycemia-induced teratogenesis is mediated by a functional deficiency of arachidonic acid. Proc Natl Acad Sci USA 82:8227–31.
93. Eriksson UJ, Dahlström E, Styrud J (1984) Metabolism and transport of nutrients in the growth-retarded and malformed offspring of diabetic rats. Diabetologia 27:272A (abstract).
94. Copeland AD, Porterfield SP (1987) Effects of streptozotocin-induced diabetes in pregnant rats on placental transport and tissue uptake of alfa-amino-isobutyric acid. Horm Metab Res 19:57–61.
95. Eriksson GL, Kihlström I, Eriksson UJ (1987) Diabetes in pregnancy: enhanced placental transport of glucose and neutral amino acids from manifest diabetic rats to their fetuses. Submitted for publication.
96. Thomas CR, Eriksson GL, Kihlström I, et al (1987) The bidirectional flux of glucose across the placenta of normal and diabetic rats. In: Renold AE, Shafrir E (eds): Lessons from Animal Diabetes II. Proceedings of the second international workshop, Geneva, Switzerland, September 9–13, 1987. John Libbey & Company Ltd, London (in press).
97. Buchanan TA, Schemmer JK, Freinkel N (1986) Embryotoxic effects of brief maternal insulin-hypoglycemia during organogenesis in the rat. J Clin Invest 78:643–9.
98. Akazawa S, Akazawa M, Yamaguchi Y, et al (1986) Effects of hypoglycemia on early embryogenesis in rat embryo organ culture. Diabetologia 29:512A (abstract).
99. Sadler TW, Hunter ES (1987) Hypoglycemia: how little is too much for the embryo? Am J Obstet Gynecol 157:190–3.
100. Ornoy A, Zusman I, Cohen AM, et al (1986) Effects of sera from Cohen, genetically determined diabetic rats, Streptozotocin diabetic rats and sucrose fed rats on *in vitro* development of early somite rat embryos. Diab Res 3:43–51.
101. Cockroft DL (1984) Abnormalities induced in cultured rat embryos by hyperglycaemia. Br J Exp Pathol 65:625–36.

102. Reece EA, Pinter E, Leranth CZ, et al (1985) Ultrastructural analysis of malformations of the embryonic neural axis induced by in vitro hyperglycemic conditions. Teratology 32:363–73.

103. Pinter E, Reece EA, Leranth CZ, et al (1986) Yolk sac failure in embryopathy due to hyperglycemia: ultrastructural analysis of yolk sac differentiation associated with embryopathy in rat conceptuses under hyperglycemic conditions. Teratology 33:73–84.

104. Brolin SE, Naeser P, Bodin B, et al (1986) Sorbitol may accumulate in early embryos, but does not seem to cause malformations. Diabetologia 29:522 (abstract).

105. Hod M, Star S, Passonneau JV, et al (1986) Effect of hyperglycemia on sorbitol and *myo*-inositol content of cultured rat conceptus: failure of aldose reductase inhibitors to modify *myo*-inositol depletion and dysmorphogenesis. Biochem Biophys Res Comm 140:974–80.

106. Pinter E, Reece EA, Leranth CA, et al (1986) Arachidonic acid prevents hyperglycemia-associated yolk sac damage and embryopathy. Am J Obstet Gynecol 155:691–702.

107. Horton WE, Sadler TW, Hunter ES (1985) Effects of hyperketonemia on mouse embryonic and fetal glucose metabolism in vitro. Teratology 31:227–33.

108. Horton WE, Sadler TW (1985) Mitochondrial alterations in embryos exposed to B-Hydroxybutyrate in whole embryo culture. Anat Rec 213:94–101.

109. Hunter ES, Sadler TW, Wynn RE (1987) A potential mechanism of DL-beta-hydroxybutyrate-induced malformations in mouse embryos. Am J Physiol 253:E72–E80.

110. Phillips LS, Fusco AC, Unterman TG (1985) Nutrition and somatomedins. XIV. Altered levels of somatomedins and somatomedin inihibitors in rats with streptozotocin-induced diabetes. Metabolism 34:765–70.

111. Sadler TW, Phillips LS, Balkan W, et al (1986) Somatomedin inhibitors from diabetic rat serum alter growth and development of mouse embryos in culture. Diabetes 35:861–5.

112. Palacin M, Lasuncion MA, Martin A, Herrera E (1985) Decreased uterine blood flow in the diabetic pregnant rat does not modify the augmented glucose transfer to the fetus. Biol Neonate 48:197–203.

113. Freinkel N, Cockroft DL, Lewis NJ, et al (1986) Fuel-mediated teratogenesis during early organogenesis: the effects of increased concentrations of glucose, ketones, or somatomedin inhibitor during rat embryo culture. Am J Clin Nutr 44:986–95.

Part II Islet Ontogeny: Fetal Pancreatic Ontogeny and Maternal Substrates

2
Adaptation of the Fetal Pancreas to Maternal Diabetes

PIERO P. FOÀ

Webster's dictionary defines a parasite as "one living at another's expense" or as "an organism living in or on another living organism obtaining from it part or all of its organic nutrients and commonly exhibiting some degree of adaptive structural modification" (1). Either definition well describes the mammalian embryo: Aristotle (2) and Leonardo da Vinci (3) knew it and so did Michele Medici, a professor at the Pontifical University of Bologna, who, about 150 years ago, wrote that "the material destined for the nutrition of the fetus is carried by the uterine blood vessels to the placenta and, after being absorbed by the latter, is transported to the fetus thanks to the umbilical vessels . . . probably without direct commerce of blood" (4). We now know that the composition of this nutritional material is the product of maternal metabolism, suitably modified by a balance of apparently opposite endocrine forces: hyperinsulinism in the fed state, albeit associated with a degree of insulin resistance, and an increased secretion of counterregulatory hormones in the fasted state (5–8). As a result of this shifting equilibrium, the mother stores nutrients during the fed state and mobilizes them during periods of fasting, thus guaranteeing an adequate and constant supply to the growing conceptus. No matter how abundant and well balanced the nutrients, to use them the embryo must develop suitable enzymes, a process regulated partly by the quality and quantity of the nutrients themselves, partly by the manner in which the nutrients are obtained, and partly by hormones that become available as gestation progresses. This endocrine and metabolic ontogeny may be divided into prenatal, neonatal, nursing, and adult periods that are marked by distinct nutritional events—that is, a switch from parenteral to oral feeding (separated by a brief period of fasting) and from a diet rich in protein and fat and relatively low in carbohydrate (milk), to one in which carbohydrate becomes the main source of calories (9–11).

In the early stages of the prenatal period, the metabolic requirements of the embryo are fulfilled by nutrients continuously supplied by the placenta, which, in the words of Claude Bernard, serves as a "transitional liver" (12). It is a "pay as you go" situation in which there is no significant accumulation of energy reserves and no evidence of pancreatic endocrine activity or of the enzymes necessary for lipogenesis and glycogen synthesis. Indeed, the first histochemically differentiated A- and B-cells appear between the eighth and tenth week of gestation. Developing at a different rate, the A-cells reach their maximum number toward the end of the second trimester of pregnancy and the B-cells approximately two months after birth; the B:A ratio increases during gestation from less than 1 to about 1 at term, to as much as 5 in the adult (10,11,13–16). Although this increase coincides with an increase in pancreatic insulin content, the mechanism for insulin release, even if demonstrable in the 32-week-old fetal pancreas (17), does not mature until the end of gestation (10,11,18), perhaps because of an inadequate production of cyclic adenosine monophosphate (cAMP) (19) or because it is restrained by an increasing number of somatostatin-secreting D-cells (20–22). The experimental conditions used to study this problem may not have been always ideal, since it is known that B-cells, even though mature, do not respond to continuous stimulation by glucose as well as they do to intermittent stimulation by a mixture of glucose and amino acids (23,24). This is especially so in the presence of a secretagogue produced by the placenta (25) and in the presence of an active enteroinsular axis (26–28). Finally, it is also possible that this "insufficiency" may not be as severe as the presumed delay in the maturation of the insulinogenic response might imply, since some of the metabolic and growth-promoting functions of insulin may be performed by the fetal pituitary growth hormone or by insulin-like growth factors produced by the placenta (29–36). In any case, maturation of the endocrine system would be of no avail unless it were accompanied by that of specific receptors and postreceptor effector mechanisms. Indeed, as gestation progress, growth hormone and placental lactogen receptors appear in the sheep, while the rat and other animals, including man develop receptors for insulin and glucagon (37–45), and many rate-limiting metabolic enzymes begin to appear in the developing liver and adipose tissue. Among these are enzymes such as uridine diphosphate glucose (UDPG)-glycosyl transferase, UDPG phosphorylase, phosphoglucomutase, malate-nicotinamide-adenine dinucleotide phosphate (NADP) dehydrogenase, and glycerokinase all necessary for the synthesis of glycogen and fat and hence for the establishment of nutritional reserves needed to prepare the fetus for the second or neonatal period of life. This period starts when placental nutrition ceases and continues until the mother produces enough milk to satisfy the needs of her baby. During this period of total or partial fasting, starvation is prevented by the glycogen and fat previously accumulated and now rapidly mobilized thanks to abrupt changes in the endocrine and enzymatic environment. Most prominent among these changes are a decrease in plasma insulin and an increased secretion of counterregulatory hormones (glucagon, catecholamines, glucocorticoids, and growth hormone), leading to a rapid decrease in the enzymes of glycogen synthesis and of lipogenesis, to a rapid increase in cAMP-dependent phosphorylase and lipase, and to a more gradual increase in gluconeogenic enzymes, such as glucose 6-phosphatase, fructose 1-6-diphosphatase, phosphoenolpyruvate carboxykinase, pyruvate carboxylase, and amino acid transaminases. The results of these changes are a rapid production of glucose from the readily available but limited reserves of liver glycogen, an increased production of lactic acid from muscle glycogen, and of fatty acid and ketones from triglycerides, followed by a sustained increase in glucose production from gluconeogenesis (10,11,46–51). The mechanism that triggers this sudden metabolic turnaround is not fully understood. Real or impending hypoglycemia and transient hypoxia may contribute by stimulating the release of glucocorticoids, glucagon, and catecholamines. These, in turn, inhibit insulin secretion and further stimulate the secretion of glucagon, either directly or through an endorphin-mediated effect (52,53).

When oral feeding becomes fully adequate, the newborn enters the third phase of metabolic adaptation in which most of the glucose continues to derive from gluconeogenesis and some from the relatively low carbohydrate content of milk. During this phase the replenishment of glycogen stores and the needs of the central nervous system and other glucose-dependent organs are protected through decreased competition with the insulin-dependent tissues whose glucose uptake is reduced by insulin resistance (54) and by the inhibitory effect of the high-fat diet (55).

The fourth and final phase begins at weaning when the dietary intake of carbohydrate increases, the endocrine system reaches full maturity, the B-cells become fully sensitive to secretagogues, glucose becomes an effective inhibitor of the A-cell, and the serum insulin to glucagon ratio increases toward the values characteristic of the adult individual.

The essential role of nutrients in the orderly development of the endocrine pancreas and fetal metabolism is further demonstrated by evidence that prenatal malnutrition, premature or delayed birth, excessive or inadequate early feeding, or the experimental alteration of the intrauterine environment can cause profound and possibly permanent endocrine, enzymatic, and metabolic changes in the offspring (10,56–60). Among these alterations are those associated with various forms of experimental or clinical diabetes, including gestational diabetes and prediabetes. In these conditions the mobilization of metabolic substrates characteristic of normal pregnancy is enhanced, and the amount of nutrients available to the fetus is increased, leading to accelerated development of the pancreatic islets, to elevated plasma insulin levels and, consequently, to fetal macrosomia and organomegaly and to neonatal hypoglycemia (61–69). This, of course, is a modified version of the hypothesis first proposed by Pedersen, who considered maternal-fetal hyperglycemia the sole prime mover (70,71) and is supported by strong experimental and clinical evidence. Thus, the fetus and the neonate of diabetic mothers often show islet hypertrophy and hyperplasia (72–75), enhanced insulin secretion, and increased levels of insulin and/or C-peptide in the amniotic fluid and in the cord blood (76–80), while the plasma insulin level of normal women is directly related to neonatal birth weight. Other causes of fetal hyperinsulinism may be stimulation of the B-cells by maternal insulin antibodies (81,82) and the transfer of maternal insulin to the fetus. This possibility cannot be excluded because although it may be safe to say that a normal placenta is impermeable to free insulin, it may be permeable to antibody-bound insulin (83). Moreover, little is known about the behavior of placentas with structural lesions due to diabetes (84). Another factor contributing to fetal macrosomia may be excessive production of somatomedin and other growth factors by the placenta (32,34,39), even though, at least in the case of somatomedin and in diabetic rats, biologic availability may be decreased by an inhibitor apparently small enough to cross the placenta (85,86). Thus, the fetus and the newborn of a diabetic mother may be exposed, on the one hand, to overfeeding, hyperinsulinism, increased number of insulin receptors, excessive growth stimulation, and neonatal hypoglycemia (61–66,87,88). On the other hand, they may be exposed to placental abnormalities, inadequate growth stimulation, and to the damaging effects of occasional episodes of maternal hypoglycemia (89–91). Although the final outcome may be determined by the severity of maternal diabetes and by the relative weight of these pathogenetic factors, all risks appear to be greatly decreased by a rigorous therapeutic regimen (92). It is not known whether, or to what extent, strict control will also reduce the probability that children of diabetic mothers will develop glucose intolerance, diabetes, or obesity later in life (93–96), or whether a diabetic fetus in any way alters the metabolism of the mother.

References

1. Gove PB (1981) Webster's Third International Dictionary of the English Language Unabridged. Merriam Co, Springfield MA.
2. Aristoteles of Stagira: On the generation of animals. Translated by Peck AL (1963) London, Cambridge MA.
3. Leonardo da Vinci, Quaderni di Anatomia. Cited by Castiglioni A (1948) Storia della Medicina Vol 1. Mondadori, Milano, p 363.
4. Medici M (1836) Manuale di Fisiologia. Tesi e Wambergher, Livorno, p 534.
5. Ward WK, Johnston CLW, Beard JC, Benedetti TG, Halter JB, Porte D Jr (1985) Insulin resistance and impaired insulin secretion in subjects with histories of gestational diabetes mellitus. Diabetes 34:861–869.
6. Toyoda N, Murata K, Sugiyama Y (1985) Insulin binding, glucose oxidation and methylglucose transport in isolated adipocytes from pregnant rats near term. Endocrinology 116:998–1002.
7. Lerario AC, Wajchenberg BL, El-Andere W, Ohnuma LY, Monaci J, Sankowsky M, Toledo E, Souza IT, Germek O (1985) Sequential studies of glucose tolerance and red blood cell insulin receptors in normal human pregnancy. Diabetes 34:780–786.

8. Hjøllund E, Pedersen O, Espersen T, Klebe JG (1986) Impaired insulin receptor binding and postbinding defects of adipocytes from normal and diabetic pregnant women. Diabetes 35:598–603.
9. Fiser RH Jr (1976) Glucose homeostasis during the perinatal period. In: New MI, Fiser RH Jr (eds) Diabetes and Other Disorders During Pregnancy and in the Newborn. Liss, New York, pp 33–50.
10. Baxter-Grillo D, Blázquez E, Grillo TAI, Sodoyez J-C, Sodoyez-Goffaux F, Foà PP (1981) Functional development of the pancreatic islets. In: Cooperstein SJ, Watkins D (eds) The Islets of Langerhans. Biochemistry, Physiology, and Pathology. Academic Press, New York, pp 35–49.
11. Ktorza A, Bihorean MT, Nurjhan N, Picon L, Girard J (1985) Insulin and glucagon during the perinatal period: secretion and metabolic effects on the liver. Biol Neonate 48:204–220.
12. Bernard C (1859) Recherches sur l'origine de la glycogénie dans la vie embryonnaire; nouvelle fonction du placenta. Compt Rend Séances Soc Biol (Paris) 1(series 3):101–107.
13. Grillo TAI, Shima K (1966) Insulin content and enzyme histochemistry of the human fetal pancreatic islet. J Endocrinol 36:151–158.
14. Rastogi GK, Letarte J, Fraser TR (1970) Immunoreactive insulin content of 103 pancreases from foetuses of healthy mothers. Diabetologia 6:445–446.
15. Wirdnam PK, Milner RDG (1981) Quantitation of the B and A cell fractions in human pancreas from early fetal life to puberty. Early Hum Dev 5:299–309.
16. Stefan Y, Grasso S, Perrelet A, Orci L (1983) A quantitative immunofluorescent study of the endocrine cell populations in the developing human pancreas. Diabetes 32:293–301.
17. Milner RDG, Leach FN, Jack PMB (1975) Reactivity of the fetal islet. In: Sutherland HW, Stowers JM (eds) Carbohydrate Metabolism in Pregnancy and the Newborn. Churchill Livingstone, Edinburgh, pp 83–104.
18. Kawazu S, Kanazawa Y, Hayashi M, Ikeuchi M, Nakai T, Kosaka K (1980) Monolayer culture of human fetal and adult pancreas. Static and dynamic studies of insulin release in vitro. Horm Metab Res 12:354–360.
19. Andersson A, Grill V, Asplund K, Berne C, Agran A, Hellerstrom C (1975) Functional maturation of the pancreatic B cell. In: Camerini-Dávalos RA, Cole HS (eds) Early Diabetes in Early Life. Academic Press, New York, pp 49–56.
20. Rahier J, Wallon J, Henquin J-C, (1981) Cell populations in the endocrine pancreas of human neonates and infants. Diabetologia 20:540–546.
21. Goldman H, Wong I, Patel YC (1982) Study of the structural and biochemical development of human fetal Islets of Langerhans. Diabetes 31:897–902.
22. Clark A, Grant AM (1983) Quantitative morphology of endocrine cells in human fetal pancreas. Diabetologia 25:31–35.
23. Grasso S, Palumbo G, Messina A, Mazzone D, Rutano G (1975) Human maternal and fetal serum insulin and growth hormone response to glucose and leucine. In: Camerini-Dávalos RA, Cole MS (eds) Early Diabetes in Early Life. Academic Press, New York, pp 537–540.
24. Sodoyez-Goffaux F, Sodoyez J-C (1976) Effects of intermittent hyperglycemia in pregnant rats on the functional development of the pancreatic B cells of their offspring. Diabetologia 12:73–76.
25. Sodoyez-Goffaux F, Sodoyez J-C, Devos CJ (1979) Insulin secretion and me-

tabolism during the perinatal period in the rat. Evidence for a placental role in fetal hyperinsulinism. J Clin Invest 63:1095–1102.

26. Oliven A, King KC, Kalhan SC (1986) Gastrointestinal enhanced insulin release in response to glucose in newborn infants. J. Pediatr Gastroenterol Nutr 5:220–225.

27. Lambert AE, Orci L, Renold AE (1970) Some factors controlling diffentiation and/or modulation of rat pancreatic islet cells. In: Camerini-Dávalos RA, Cole HS (eds) Early Diabetes. Academic Press, New York, pp 35–43.

28. Lucas A (1986) Breastfeeding and gut hormones. In: Filer LJ Jr, Fomon SJ (eds) The Breastfed Infant: A Model of Performance. 91st Ross Conf Ped Res, Ross Laboratories, Columbus OH, pp 73–87.

29. Blázquez E, Simon FA, Blázques M, Foà PP (1974) Changes in serum growth hormone levels from fetal to adult age in the rat. Proc Soc Exp Biol Med 147:780–783.

30. Ashton IK, Zapf J, Einschenk TJ, MacKenzie IZ (1985) Insulin-like growth factors (IGF) 1 and 2 in human fetal plasma and relationship to gestational age and fetal size during midpregnancy. Acta Endocrinol (Copenh) 110:558–563.

31. Bennett A, Wilson DM, Lin F, Nagashima R, Rosenfeld RG, Hintz RL (1983) Levels of insulin-like growth factors I and II in human cord blood. J Clin Endocrinol Metab 57:609–612.

32. Lin K-S, Wang C-Y, Mills N, Gyves M, Ilan J (1985) Insulin-related genes expressed in human placenta from normal and diabetic pregnancies. Proc Natl Acad Sci USA 82:3868–3870.

33. Underwood LE, D'Ercole AJ (1984) Insulin and insulin-like growth factors/somatomedins in fetal and neonatal development. J Clin Endocrinol Metab 13:69–89.

34. Chernausek SD, Chatelain PG, Svoboda ME, Underwood LE, Van Wyk JJ (1985) Efficient purification of somatomedin C/insulin-like growth factor I using immunoaffinity chromatography. Biochem Biophys Res Commun 126:282–288.

35. Hill DJ, Milner RDG (1985) Insulin as a growth factor. Pediatr Res 19:879–886.

36. Sheppard MS, Bala RM (1986) Profile of serum immunoreactive insulin-like growth factor I during gestation in Wistar rats. Can J Physiol Pharmacol 64:521–524.

37. Fant M, Munro H, Moses AC (1986) An autocrine/paracrine role for insulin-like growth factors in the regulations of human placental growth. J Clin Endocrinol Metab 63:499–505.

38. Freemark M, Comer M, Handwergen S (1986) Placental lactogen and GH receptors in sheep liver: striking differences in ontogeny and function. Am J Physiol 251:E328–E333.

39. Blázquez E, Rubalcava B, Montesano R, Orci L, Unger RH (1976) Development of insulin and glucagon binding and the adenylate cyclase response in liver membranes of the prenatal, postnatal and adult rat: evidence of glucagon "resistance". Endocrinology 98:1014–1023.

40. Thorsson AV, Hintz RL (1977) Insulin receptors in the newborn. Increase in receptor affinity and number. N Engl J Med 297:908–912.

41. Kappy MS, Plotnick LP, Milley JR, Rosenberg A, Molteni RA, Jones MD Jr,

Simmons MA (1981) Ontogeny of erythrocyte insulin binding in the sheep. Endocrinology 109:611–617.
42. Vinicor F, Kiedrowski L (1982) Characterization of the hepatic receptor for insulin in the perinatal rat. Endocrinology 110:782–790.
43. Ganguli S, Sinha M, Sperling MA (1984) Ontogeny of insulin and glucagon receptors and the adenylate cyclase system in guinea pig liver. Pediatr Res 18:558–565.
44. Morriss FH Jr, Tuchman C, Crandell SS, Riddle LM, Fitzgerald BJ, West MS (1986) Ontogeny of ovine fetal liver and kidney plasma membrane insulin receptors and fetal growth. Proc Soc Exp Biol Med 181:24–32.
45. Unterman T, Goewert RR, Baumann G, Freinkel N (1986) Insulin receptors in embryo and extra-embryonic membranes of early somite rat conceptus. Diabetes 35:1193–1199.
46. Greengard O (1975) Enzymatic differentiation during hepatic development. In: Camerini-Dávalos RA, Cole HS (eds) Early Diabetes in Early Life. Academic Press, New York pp 9–14.
47. Shelley HJ, Bassett JM, Milner RDG (1975) Control of carbohydrate metabolism in the fetus and newborn. Br Med Bull 31:37–43.
48. Cuezva JM, Valcarce C, Medina JM (1985) Substrates availability for maintenance of energy homeostasis in the immediate postnatal period of the fasted newborn rat. In: Jonas CT, Nathanielsz PW (eds) The Physiological Development of the Fetus and Newborn. Academic Press, New York pp 63–69.
49. Räihä NCR (1979) Hormonal regulation of perinatal enzyme differentiation in the mammalian liver. In: Elliott K, O'Connor M (eds) Pregnancy Metabolism, Diabetes and the Fetus. Ciba Found Symp 63, Excerpta Med, Amsterdam pp 137–160.
50. Ruiz-Bravo N, Ernest MJ (1985) Multihormonal control of tyrosine aminotransferase activity in developing rat liver. Endocrinology 116:2489–2496.
51. Denne SC, Kalhan SC (1986) Glucose carbon recycling and oxidation in human newborns. Am J Physiol 251:E71–E77.
52. Helman AM, Giraud P, Nicolaidis S, Oliver C, Assan R (1983) Glucagon release after stimulation of the lateral hypothalamic area in rats: predominant β-adrenergic transmission and involvement of endorphin pathways. Endocrinology 113:1–6.
53. Stark RI, Wardlaw SL, Daniel SS (1986) Characterization of plasma β-endorphin immunoreactivity in the fetal lamb: effects of gestational age and hypoxia. Endocrinology 119:755–761.
54. Blázquez E, Lipshaw LA, Blázquez M, Foà PP (1975) The synthesis and release of insulin in fetal, nursing and young adult rats: studies in vivo and in vitro. Pediatr Res 9:17–25.
55. Begum N, Tepperman HM, Tepperman J (1985) Insulin-induced internalization and replacement of insulin receptors in adipocytes of rats adapted to fat feeding. Diabetes 34:1272–1277.
56. Schwartz R, Susa J (1980) Fetal macrosomia. Animal models. Diabetes Care 3:430–432.
57. Freinkel N, Lewis NJ, Johnson R, Swenne R, Bone A, Hellerstrom C (1984) Differential effects of age versus glycemic stimulation on the maturation of insulin stimulus-secretion coupling during culture of fetal rat islet. Diabetes 33:1028–1038.

58. Russell G, Dawodu AK, Shennan AT (1984) Glucose homeostasis in the heavy-for-date neonate. In: Sutherland HW, Stowers JM (eds) Carbohydrate Metabolism in Pregnancy and the Newborn. Churchill Livingstone, Edinburgh, pp 150–151.
59. Cella SG, Locatelli V, de Gennaro V, Puggioni R, Pintor C, Müller EE (1985) Human pancreatic growth hormone (GH)-releasing hormone stimulates GH synthesis and release in infant rats. An in vivo study. Endocrinology 116:574–577.
60. Domenech M, Gruppuso PA, Susa JB, Schwartz T (1985) Induction in utero of hepatic glucose 6-phosphatase by fetal hypoinsulinemia. Biol Neonate 47:92–98.
61. Szabo AJ, Szabo O (1974) Placental free-fatty-acid transfer and fetal adipose tissue development: an explanation of fetal adiposity in infants of diabetic mothers. Lancet II:498–499.
62. Freinkel N (1980) The Banting Lecture 1980: Of pregnancy and progeny. Diabetes 29:1023–1035.
63. Metzger BE, Phelps RL, Freinkel N, Navikas IA (1980) Effects of gestational diabetes on diurnal profiles of plasma glucose, lipids, and individual amino acids. Diabetes Care 3:402–409.
64. Freinkel N, Dooley SL, Metzger BE (1985) Care of the pregnant woman with insulin-dependent diabetes mellitus. N Engl J Med 313:96–101.
65. Freinkel N, Metzger BE, Phelps RL, Simpson JL, Martin AO, Radvany R, Ober C, Dooley SL, Depp RO, Belton A (1986) Gestational diabetes mellitus: a syndrome with phenotypic and genotypic heterogeneity. Horm Metab Res 18:427–430.
66. Heding LG, Persson B, Stangenberg M (1980) B-cell function in newborn infants of diabetic mothers. Diabetologia 19:427–432.
67. Tallarigo L, Giampietro O, Penno G, Miccoli R, Gregori G, Navalesi R (1986) Relation of glucose tolerance to complications of pregnancy in nondiabetic women. N Engl J Med 315:984–992.
68. Philipps AF, Rosenkrantz TS, Grunnet ML, Connolly ME, Porte PJ, Raye JR (1986) Effects of fetal insulin secretory deficiency on metabolism in fetal lamb. Diabetes 35:964–972.
69. Freinkel N, Metzger BE (1979) Pregnancy as a tissue culture experience: the critical implications of maternal metabolism for fetal development. In: Elliott K, O'Connor M (eds) Pregnancy Metabolism, Diabetes and the Fetus. Ciba Found Symp 63, Excerpta Med, Amsterdam pp 3–28.
70. Pedersen J (1952) Diabetes and Pregnancy. Blood Sugar of Newborn Infants. A thesis. Danish Science Press, Copenhagen.
71. Pedersen J (1967) The pregnant diabetic and her newborn. Problems and management. Munksgaard, Copenhagen, pp 219.
72. Dubrueil G, Anderodias J (1920) Ilôts de Langerhans géants chez un nouveau-né issu de mère glycosurique. Compt Rend Séances Soc Biol (Paris) 83:1490–1493.
73. Van Assche FA (1975) The fetal endocrine pancreas. In: Sutherland HW, Stowers JM (eds) Carbohydrate Metabolism in Pregnancy and the Newborn. Churchill Livingstone, Edinburgh, pp 68–82.
74. Milner RDG, Wirdnam, PK, Tsanakas Y (1981) Quantitative morphology of B, A, D and PP cells in infants of diabetic mothers. Diabetes 30:271–274.

75. v Dorsche HH, Reiher H, Hahn H-J (1984) Quantitativ-histolgische Unter-suchugen des fetalen menschlichen Pankreas von stoffwechselgesunden Frauen und insulinabhängingen Diabetikerinnen. Acta Anat 118:139–143.
76. Hill DE (1979) Effect of insulin on fetal growth. In: Merkatz IR, Adam PAJ (eds) The Diabetic Pregnancy. A Perinatal Perspective. Grune & Stratton, New York, pp 155–165.
77. Heding LG, Persson B, Stangenberg M (1980) B-cell function in newborn infants of diabetic mothers. Diabetologia 19:427–432.
78. Reiher H, Fuhrmann K, Noack S, Besch W, Hahn H-J (1984) The in vitro insulin secretion of human fetal pancreatic slices from diabetic and non-diabetic women. A methodical study. Exp Clin Endocrinol 83:110–112.
79. Freinkel N, Metzger BE, Phelps RL, Dooley SL, Ogata ES, Radvany RM, Belton A (1985) Gestational diabetes mellitus. Heterogeneity of maternal age, weight, insulin secretion, HLA antigen and islet cell antibodies and the impact of maternal metabolism in pancretic B-cell and somatic development in the offspring. Diabetes 34(suppl 2):1–7.
80. Shima K, Price S, Foà PP (1966) Serum insulin concentration and birth weight in human infants. Proc Soc Exp Biol Med 121:55–59.
81. Lacy PE, Wright PH (1965) Allergic interstitial pancreatitis in rats injected with guinea pig anti-insulin serum. Diabetes 14:634–642.
82. Klöppel G, Freytag G, Bommer G (1972) Enzymehistochemical studies on the pancreatic islets in mice injected with anti-insulin serum. Diabetologia 8:19–28.
83. Roth J, Kahn CR, King GL, Meggesi K (1979) Receptors in infants of diabetic mothers. In: Cornblath M, Kaye R, Little B, Segal S (eds) Workshop on Fetal Development in the Infant of the Diabetic Mother. Juvenile Diabetes Found pp 28–40.
84. Haust MD (1981) Maternal diabetes mellitus. Effects on the fetus and placenta. In: Naeye RL, Kissane JM, Kaufman N (eds) Perinatal Diseases. Williams & Wilkins, Baltimore, pp 201–285.
85. Phillips LS, Vassilopoulou-Sellin R, Reichard LA (1979) Nutrition and so-matomedin. VIII. The ''somatomedin inhibitor'' in diabetic rat serum is a gen-eral inhibitor of growing cartilage. Diabetes 28:919–924.
86. Sadler TW, Phillips LS, Balkan W, Goldstein S (1986) Somatomedin inhibitors from diabetic rat serum alter growth and development of mouse embryos in culture. Diabetes 35:861–865.
87. Cornblath M, Pildes RS, Warrner RA (1970) Infants of the diabetic mother. In: Camerini-Dávalos RA, Cole HS (eds): Early Diabetes. Academic Press, New York, pp 241–252.
88. Neufeld ND, Corbo LM (1986) Insulin-receptor development in normal and diabetic pregnancies. Role of membrane fluidity. Diabetes 35:1020–1026.
89. Gewolb IH, Merdian W, Warshaw JB, Enders AC (1986) Fine structural ab-normalities of the placenta in diabetic rats. Diabetes 35:1254–1261.
90. Heinze E, Brenner R, Nguyen-Thi Ch, Vetter U, Leupold D, Pohlandt F (1986) Skeletal growth in fetal rats. Effects of glucose and amino acids. Diabetes 35:222–227.
91. Buchanan TA, Schemmer JK, Freinkel N (1986) Embryotoxic effects of brief maternal insulin-hypoglycemia during organogenesis in the rat. J Clin Invest 78:643–649.

92. Fuhrmann K, Reiher H, v Dorsche HH (1985) Hyperinsulinemia in the fetus of the diabetic mother. Is prevention possible? In: Serano-Rios M, Lefèbvre PJ (eds) Diabetes 1985. Excerpta Med, Amsterdam, pp 598–603.
93. Farquhar JW (1969) The infant of the diabetic mother. Postgrad Med J 45:806–811.
94. Shah MPK, Farquhar JW (1975) Children of diabetic mothers. Subsequent weight. In: Camerini-Dávalos RA, Cole HS (eds), Early Diabetes in Early Life. Academic Press, New York, pp 587–593.
95. Bihoreau MT, Ktorza A, Kinebanyan MF, Picon L (1986) Impaired glucose homeostasis in adult rats from hyperglycemic mothers. Diabetes 35:979–984.
96. Abbott WGH, Thuillez P, Howard BV, Salans LB, Cushman SW, Reaven GW, Foley JE (1986) Body composition, adipocyte size, free fatty acid concentration and glucose tolerance in children of diabetic pregnancies. Diabetes 35:1077–1080.

3
The Use of Human Fetal Pancreatic Tissue for Transplantation

CHARLES M. PETERSON, LOIS JOVANOVIC, AND BENT FORMBY

History

The idea of using fetal pancreata as a source of insulin-secreting tissue is not new. A number of investigators, including Banting and Best, have favored the use of fetal tissue at one time or another, citing the relative lack of development of exocrine tissue and hence the relative abundance of endocrine cells with lessened possibility of enzymatic digestion of insulin or insulin-containing cells (1). In 1928 the human fetal pancreas was first used for tranplantation purposes (2). In that year Fichera placed pancreatic tissue from three fetuses into various sites in an 18-year-old man with diabetes mellitus. The experiment failed in that the recipient died in a diabetic coma three days later.

Despite these inauspicious beginnings, there was a resurgence of interest in the procedure of fetal islet or whole pancreas transplantation starting in about 1977. The impetus for this renewed consideration of an abandoned procedure lay in the high morbidity and mortality associated with vascularized transplants in man and in the experiments of Sutherland (3) and of Brown and co-workers (4,5), which documented that implantation of fetal rat pancreas could reverse experimental diabetes in adult animals. At the present time, perhaps as many as 400 transplants of fetal pancreatic tissue into man have taken place, mostly in the People's Republic of China and the Soviet Union (6–8).

Studies of Isolation, Storage, Shipment, and Function In vitro

Kemp et al (9) and Dr. Brown's group (10) were also the first to demonstrate that the histologically complex rodent fetal pancreas could be stored indefinitely in the frozen state and successfully used to reverse diabetes after transplantation and that such an approach might be applicable to humans. Since that time a great deal of effort in a number of laboratories has been devoted to the study of the optimum source and handling of potentially transplantable human fetal tissue. Such studies are particularly important since the β-cell content of a single human fetal pancreas is not inherently sufficient to normalize the hyperglycemia of an adult diabetic recipient. Therefore, successful transplantation must either await significant expansion and differentiation of the implanted fetal β-cell mass or material collected from more than one fetus needs to be implanted in a single procedure.

Quantitative immunofluorescence studies of the endocrine cell content in the developing human pancreas (11) have also shown that eight- to ten-week fetuses have a sizeable population of endocrine cells of which almost 50% react solely with antibody to glicentin (a proglucagon peptide). It is not known whether such cells represent transitional cells or α-cell precursors (12). Somatostatin-containing cells are the second most abundant endocrine cells from the 17th week of gestation up to the fifth postnatal month, but become the least numerous in the adult (13). As gestation advances, β-cell mass increases and the insulin to glucagon ratio rises from 1.5 at 20 to 24 weeks to 5 in newborn infants (14). At all fetal ages the number of islets isolated from the splenic half of the pancreas is greater than that of the duodenal half (15).

Prior to this decade, research on the fetal pancreas was limited by the lack of available tissue. Since the founding of the National Disease Research Interchange (NDRI) in Philadelphia, Pennsylvania, the availability of tissue for study has become less of a problem. Any qualified investigator may now apply for tissue through the NDRI.

We have found that tissue obtained immediately after dilation and extraction procedures and placed in ice-cold RPMI 1640 culture medium containing 20 mmol/L Hepes and glutamine at pH 7.4 gives the best results. Viability can be assessed in two ways: by trypan blue exclusion and by analysis of the insulin secretory capacity (16–19).

In our laboratory the pancreata are dissected aseptically from the surrounding tissue, stored in ice-cold sterile RPMI 1640 culture medium (Gibco) containing 20 mmol/L Hepes and 10% fetal calf serum, pH 7.4, chopped into fine fragments (1 to 2 mm), and digested in warm (38 °C) magnesium-free Hanks' buffered salt solution (HBSS) containing 7 mg/mL collagenase (Sigma grade V), 5 mmol/L glucose, and 1% human albumin for 75 minutes in an agitator water bath (shaking at the rate of 120 c/min). The digest is then washed three times with ice-cold HBSS and samples of 100- to 300-μm islets are selected under a microscope and transferred to nontissue petri dishes and incubated for 48 hours at 37 °C in 95% air/5% CO_2 with RPMI 1640 supplemented with 10% human adult serum. About 800 to 1,500 islets are isolated from each donor pancreas and are incubated in separate dishes.

To analyze staining with trypan blue, fetal islets are incubated in a 0.04% solution of the dye in isotonic Krebs-Ringer buffer (KRB) pH 7.40 for 15 minutes, carefully washed several times in KRB, and counted under a microscope. The percentage of unstained islets can then be calculated and/or viable islets selected by hand.

Insulin release in response to glucose stimulation is measured in two successive one-hour static incubations. After culture and staining, islets isolated from each fetal pancreas are transferred to plastic tubes and incubated in KRB, pH 7.4, containing 25 mmol/L Hepes, 2 mmol/L glucose, and 0.3% bovine serum albumin (BSA) at 37 °C in an atmosphere of 95% O_2/5% CO_2. After a first period of one hour to stabilize basal secretion, buffer is removed and a fresh KRB solution containing sufficient glucose to bring the total concentration to 25 mmol/L with or without 1 mmol/L 3-isobutyl-1-methyl-xanthine (IBMX) as a potentiator is added and the islets are reincubated for an additional hour. After each incubation, samples of the buffer are removed for radioimmunoassay of insulin, using human insulin as reference standard. Insulin remaining within the islets at the end of the second static incubation is extracted with acidic ethanol and assayed. The fractional-stimulated insulin secretion rate is defined as the amount of insulin released during the second hour of incubation and expressed as a percentage of total insulin content taken as the sum of the insulin secreted during the second hour plus the final nonsecreted insulin content at the end of the experiment.

Using this protocol, we have determined that fetal pancreatic tissue remains viable under conditions of cold storage at 0 to 2 °C for up to 144 hours, although warming adversely effects survival. These observations indicate that the tissue can be shipped packed in ice, which markedly enhances the potential usefulness of this tissue. Up to 144 hours of culture after 18 hours of cold storage also did not adversely affect islet viability. Finally, the insulin secretory response to glucose, while sluggish when compared with that of the adult pancreas, was found to be a function of gestational age, with relative insulin secretory capacity decreasing to a nadir at 20 to 23 weeks and gradually increasing again thereafter. These latter findings may have implications for the development of macrosomia, since glucose intolerance before 18 weeks may initiate excess insulin secretion in the fetus despite normal maternal glucose levels during the second trimester and beyond.

As documented recently by Sandler et al (20), the proliferative capacity of human fetal pancreatic cells in culture greatly depends on the condition and handling of the donor tissue. Thus, there is a wide variation in the viability of donor tissue as assessed both histologically and by growth in culture, depending on how the tissue was obtained, stored, and cultured. The optimum handling of fetal islet tissue and the optimum environment for storage and induction of proliferation remain to be determined.

The technique described above was modified slightly from that of Ågren et al (21), who used pancreatic fragments that were transferred to non-attachment sterile culture dishes containing either 5 mL tissue culture medium (TCM) 199 or RPMI 1640 supplemented with 10% to 20% fetal calf serum and antibiotics. The cultures were maintained at 37 °C in an atmosphere of 5%. CO_2 in humidified air. With this procedure the fragments remain unattached by resting on the bottom of the dishes, thereby creating some gas diffusion problems in the fairly large cellular fragments. These investigators found that after six to 14 days in culture, the fragments were composed of fibrous tissue, well-preserved ducts and islet cells, some of which were organized into islets, whereas acinar cells seemed to have disappeared. Insulin-release experiments demonstrated that a high glucose concentration alone failed to stimulate insulin secretion; however, the addition of 5 mmol/L theophylline to 15 mmol/L glucose did elicit a slight to marked insulin response from the cultured pancreatic fragments. No difference in the secretory response was observed between islets cultured in TCM 199 and in RPMI 1640. These investigators could not document a correlation between stimulated insulin release and fetal age.

Another method uses tissue fragments cultured on a raft in order to maintain the tissue at the gas-medium interface (22,23). The respiring tissue is provided with optimal gas exchange and access to the nutrients of the culture medium. Andersson et al (23) used cultured minced fragments on Millipore filters supported by surgical gel foam in the presence of either medium RPMI 1640 or TCM 199 and found a considerable decrease in the insulin accumulation in the culture medium when explants were maintained in RPMI 1640 but not in TCM 199. Nevertheless, a comparison between the air-liquid interface techniques and the free-floating suspension failed to demonstrate a clearcut difference between the two methods with regard to insulin output.

Using a similar culture technique, Maitland and co-workers reported that their fetal explants responded with augmented insulin release to either 1.5μmol/L glucagon, 5 mmol/L leucine, 10 mmol/L arginine, or 10 mmol/L theophylline and only slightly to 19.3 mmol/L glucose (24). Elevation of the glucose concentration in TCM 199 seemed to maintain a higher insulin secretion in the cultures. Addition of an amino acid mixture also enhanced the insulin secretion of human fetal pancreatic explants in culture (25). Maitland et al furthermore found that a high oxygen concentration (95% O_2 and 5% CO_2) was toxic to the explants and suggested a gas phase of air plus 5% CO_2 (26). A toxic effect of high O_2 concentration was reported also by Mandel and Koulmanda (27) in experiments designed to decrease the immunogenicity of fetal mouse pancreas before allogeneic transplantation. Our unpublished observations concur with these findings on the effects of high oxygen.

Sandler et al (20), recently described a method for the culture of human fetal pancreas in which islet-like cell clusters (ICC), partly composed of endocrine cells, gradually develop in vitro. RPMI 1640 is used as the culture medium, and different biologic supplements, such as fetal calf serum, human amniotic fluid, and human serum have been tested for their effects on growth and function of the endocrine cells (20,28,29). In the presence of either human amniotic fluid, or human serum, the ICC became more abundant, but smaller and free-floating, than those cultured in the presence of fetal calf serum. In the latter medium, ICC were attached to a confluent monolayer of fibroblasts growing on the bottom of the culture dishes. A similar observation was made by Goldman and Colle (30). We have confirmed these observations. We have found also that the addition of human recombinant growth hormone increases insulin output in vitro and increases intracellular insulin messenger RNA (31). It has previously been documented in the rat that growth hormone stimulates islet β-cell replication in monolayer cultures (32). It would appear that the human fetal islet is highly sensitive to a number of growth factors in vitro and that the ontogeny of this tissue is rapidly being defined.

Cryopreservation of fetal islet tissue for potential transplantation is also a possibility as noted previously (10). Sandler and co-workers have recently documented that these techniques can by used with human fetal pancreatic tissue as well (33), thus confirming the work of Kemp et al (34).

Studies of Function In vivo

Xenografts

The availability of the immunosuppressed nude (Nu/Nu) mouse has provided investigators with the opportunity to study xenografted tissue without the administration of toxic immunosuppressive drugs. Transplantation of ICC that had been cultured beneath the kidney capsule of nude mice has been described (20). Eight weeks after transplantation, the recipient mice were injected with ^{3}H-thymidine one hour before sacrifice. In seven of nine animals receiving transplants, histologic sections from the graft showed pseudoislets composed of β- or α-cells and surrounded by non-stained epithelioid cells. There were also duct-like structures composed of occasional hormone positive cells. The number and proportion of β-cells increased in the grafted ICC as compared with the nongrafted ones examined five days after culture. The labeling index for the entire cell population in the grafts was about five times higher than the corresponding values for islets prepared from adult mice.

These findings are in good agreement with those of Tuck and co-workers, who demonstrated a histologic differentiation of endocrine cells occurring in vivo after implantation (35), although this group had some difficulty in making nude mice of different strains diabetic, in contrast to other groups who had little difficulty in this regard (36,37). Initially, Tuck and co-workers placed both fresh and cultured human fetal pancreatic slices into the subcutaneous space of diabetic nude mice. The explants coalesced soon after transplantation, becoming visible within two weeks as the scar tissue regressed. Thereafter the implants grew visibly for at least 37 weeks. Growth was inversely related to the time the tissue was cultured before transplantation, most growth occurring in uncultured tissue. In all cases when explants were cultured for up to 3 weeks prior to transplantation, tissue was macroscopically visible. In contrast, tissue cultured for longer periods could rarely be seen. Experiments in mice that were not diabetic demonstrated that uncultured subcutaneous implants would continue to grow for up to 54 weeks (38), indicating a possible adverse affect of the diabetic environment per se. In these latter experiments, a linear relationship was demonstrated between the total age of the implant (gestational age + age of the implant in the nude mouse) and its wet weight. The maximum weight reached by an implant was 730 mg. The investigators concluded that the limiting factor for the growth of human fetal tissue in nude mice was more likely to be the life span of the mouse than an intrinsic factor in the tissue itself. Insulin content of the tissue correlated with morphometric quantitation of islet cell content in the transplant tissue.

Thus human fetal pancreatic tissue implanted into nude mice appears to differentiate into endocrine tissue, ducts, and fibrous tissue. Exocrine tissue has not been identified in the implants. These findings have been observed in both diabetic and nondiabetic mice and whether the tissue was implanted into peripheral or central sites, as reported by Tuch and co-workers as well as others (39–41).

Both Tuch and colleagues, and Noonan and co-workers have been able to demonstrate normalization of blood glucose following implantation of human fetal pancreatic tissue into diabetic nude mice (42,43). However, removal of the implanted tissue did not generally result in a relapse, suggesting that the mouse pancreas had regenerated, as it sometimes does in the streptozotocin diabetic animal (44).

Allografts

The above studies led to renewed interest in the use of human fetal islet tissue transplants as a potential treatment of type I diabetes mellitus in man. The group in Uppsala, Sweden, has transplanted human pancreatic tissue in six individuals since 1979. All were insulin dependent and also had received a kidney transplant and thus were already receiving immunosuppression. Three patients who received transplants of pancreatic fragments and one who received a suspension of islets by intraportal injection had urinary C-peptide levels 5% of normal. After 4 months, the C-peptide production ceased. Interestingly, when the urinary C-peptide disappeared, the patient exhibited antibodies against islet cell surface antigen. In the other two patients there was no evidence of graft function.

In 1982 one patient received, intraportally, transplants of cryopreserved human fetal pancreatic fragments from 24 donors. Two additional patients received injections of ICC, which had developed in culture in the presence of fetal calf serum. In one of the patients the material was given intraportally as a single injection; in the other patient an indwelling catheter was used for repeated intraportal injections over a period of 6 weeks. In none of these patients were there any signs of graft function (45,28).

Clinical transplants of human fetal pancreas commenced in Sydney, Australia, in 1983 and to date five C-peptide negative patients have received human fetal tissue. All patients but one received immunosuppressive treatment with cyclosporine (cyclosporin-A), prednisone, azathioprine, and/or antilymphocyte globulin and received tissue from one to six fetal pancreata of gestational ages varying between 14 and 20 weeks. The tissue was transplanted either into the omentum or muscle tissue and was typed for histocompatibility antigens A, B, and OR (46). In only two patients who received tissue from six donors was C-peptide detected after a glucagon challenge, and in one patient it was accompanied by a 50% drop in insulin requirement. It should be noted that this latter patient had a normal glucosylated hemoglobin value prior to transplantation. Since the patient received implants at multiple sites, it was impossible to determine which implant was responsible for the C-peptide secretion. From these experiments the investigators concluded that multiple donors are needed for effective transplantation (47,48).

To date, we have implanted four C-peptide negative patients with fetal pancreatic fragments obtained from six to 12 donors. Initially, the tissue was implanted into the brachioradialis of the nondominant forearm. However, in order to find an easily accessible site with more room, in the second two recipients the tissue was transplanted into a pocket of the rectus abdominus in the left lower quadrant. In each case, exogenous insulin was given by continuous subcutaneous insulin infusion to normalize blood glucose values, documented by home glucose monitoring and glucosylated hemoglobin levels. Immunosuppression was not used. In each case C-peptide levels following a "Sustacal" (mixed protein, fat, and carbohydrate meal) challenge were detected within 3 weeks following implantation and have remained detectable for up to a year afterwards. All patients required insulin to maintain normoglycemia (19).

Conclusions and Implications for the Infant of the Woman With Diabetes Mellitus

These studies document that fetal islet tissue can be obtained, stored, cultured, and transplanted into rodents and man. In some cases, following transplantation into man, the tissue may remain viable and secrete insulin for varying periods of time. Nevertheless, thus far the clinical results have been erratic, and the development of optimum techniques to attain insulin independence in the transplant recipient requires further study.

Although the use of fetal islets for transplantation purposes remains a tantalizing but unfulfilled goal, much has been learned about the potential relevance of this tissue to the diabetic woman and her offspring. The sensitivity of fetal tissue to glucose and a number of growth factors as early as 13 weeks indicates a vulnerability of this tissue to perturbations in glucose homeostasis at a much earlier stage in gestation than was previously thought. The rapid response of this tissue (hours to days) to changes in culture conditions also has implications in terms of the response to the reestablishment of the normal maternal/fetal metabolic milieu and its potentially beneficial effect on fetal development. If, as has been suggested, pregnancy is a "tissue culture experience" (49), then studies of the human fetal pancreas as a potential transplant tissue are especially worthy of attention for the individual interested in the field of diabetes and pregnancy.

References

1. Bliss M (1982) The Discovery of Insulin. Chicago, The University of Chicago Press, pp 28–29.
2. Downing R (1984) Historical review of pancratic islet transplantation. World J Surg 8:137–142.
3. Sutherland DER (1981) Pancreas and islet transplantation: II Clinical trials. Diabetologia 20:435–450.
4. Brown J, Clark WR, Molnar IG, Mullen YS (1976) Fetal pancreas transplantation for reversal of streptozotocin-induced diabetes in rats. Diabetes 25:56–64.
5. Brown J, Molnar IG, Clark W, Mullen Y (1974) Control of experimental diabetes mellitus in rats by transplantation of fetal pancreases. Science 184:1377–1379.
6. Sutherland DER, Goetz FC, Najarian JS (1981) Review of world's experience with pancreas and islet transplantation and results of intraperitoneal segmental pancreas transplantation from related and cadaver donors at Minnesota. Transplant Proc 13:291–297.
7. Hu Y-F (1985) Clinical studies on islet transplantation in 39 patients with insulin-dependent (type I) diabetes mellitus. Wuhan Int Symp Organ Transplant 39–40.
8. Shumakov VI, Bljumkin VN, Ignatenko SN, et al (1986) The principal results of pancreatic islet cell culture transplantation in diabetes mellitus patients. Int Congress Transplant Soc 11:40.
9. Kemp JA, Mullen Y, Weisman H, et al (1978) Reversal of diabetes in rats using fetal pancreases stored at − 196 °C. Transplantation 26:260–264.
10. Brown J, Kemp JA, Hurt S, et al (1980) Cryopreservation of human fetal pancreas. Diabetes 29 [Suppl 1]:170–73.
11. Stefan Y, Grasso S, Perrelet A, et al (1983) A quantitative immunofluorescent study of the endocrine cell populations in the developing human pancreas. Diabetes 32:293–301.

12. Stefan Y, Ravazzola M, Grasso S, et al (1982) Glicentin precedes glucagon in the developing human pancreas. Endocrinology 110:2189–2191.
13. Orci L, Stefan Y, Malaisse-Lagae F, et al (1979) Instability of pancreatic endocrine cell populations throughout life. Lancet 1:615–616.
14. Wirdnam PK, Milner RDG (1981) Quantitation of the B and A cell fractions in human pancreas from early fetal life to puberty. Early Hum Dev 5:299–309.
15. Goldman H, Wong I, Patel YC (1982) A study of the structural and biochemical development of human fetal islets of Langerhans. Diabetes 31:897–902.
16. Formby B, Walker L, Peterson CM (1985) Improved isolation yield of murine islets of Langerhans from a single donor can reverse experimental diabetes after isotransplantation. Diabetes Res 2:217–219.
17. Formby B, Walker L, Peterson CM (1986) Rapid selection of viable transplantable human fetal pancreatic islets by trypan blue exclusion. Proc Soc Exp Biol Med 182:245–247.
18. Peterson CM, Miller N, Walker L, Formby B (1986) Effect of glipizide on insulin secretion from cultured human fetal pancreatic islets. Diabetes Care 9:556–557.
19. Peterson CM, Jovanovic L, Formby B, Fuhrman K, Walker L, Brennan M, and Rashbaum Wm (1986) Studies of human fetal pancreas. Proceedings of the Second International Conference on the Use of Human Tissues and Organs for Research and Transplant. National Diabetes Research Interchange, Philadelphia, Pa. pp 220–222.
20. Sandler S, Andersson A, Schnell A, et al (1985) Tissue culture of human fetal pancreas. Development and function of B-cells *in vitro* and transplantation of explants to nude mice. Diabetes 34:1113–1119.
21. Ågren A, Andersson A, Bjorken C, et al (1980) Human fetal pancreas. Culture and function in vitro. Diabetes 29 [Suppl 1]:64–69.
22. Auerbach R (1960) Morphogenetic interactions in the development t of the mouse thymus gland. Dev Biol 2:271–284.
23. Andersson A, Christensen N, Groth C-G, et al (1984) Survivial of human fetal pancreatic explants in organ culture as reflected in insulin secretion and oxygen consumption. Transplantation 37:499–503.
24. Maitland JE, Parry DG, Turtle JR (1980) Perifusion and culture of human fetal pancreas. Diabetes 29 [Suppl 1]:57–63.
25. Hoffman L, Mandel TE, Carter WM, et al (1982) Insulin secretion by fetal human pancreas in organ culture. Diabetologia 23:426–430.
26. Maitland JE, Caterson ID, Gauci RE, et al (1985) Organ culture of human foetal pancreas: Conditions which affect basal and stimulated insulin release. Acta Endocrinol 108:377–385.
27. Mandel TE, Koulmanda M (1984) Effect of cultue conditions on fetal mouse pancreas in vitro and after transplantation in syngeneic and allogeneic recipients. Diabetes 34:1082–1087.
28. Sandler S, Andersson A, Swenne I, et al (1987) Tissue culture and cryopreservation of fetal mammalian endocrine pancreas intended for transplantation. In: Peterson CM, Jovanovic L, Formby B (eds) Human Fetal Islet Transplantation. Springer Verlag, New York (in press).
29. Andersson A, Sandler S, Hellerstrom C, et al (1986) Effects of amniotic fluid on the development of human fetal pancreatic B-cells in tissue culture. Transplant Proc 18:57–59.

30. Goldman H, Colle E (1976) Human pancreatic islets in culture: Effects of supplementing the medium with homologous and heterologous serum. Science 192:1014–1016.
31. Formby B, Ullrich A, Coussens L, et al (1987) Transcriptional regulation of human fetal insulin gene expression by recombinant growth hormone. In Preparation.
32. Rabinovitch A, Quigley C, Rechler MM (1983) Growth hormone stimulates islet B-cell replication in neonatal rat pancreatic monolayer cultures. Diabetes 32:307–312.
33. Sandler S, Andersson A, Hellerstrom C, et al (1982) Preservation of morphology, insulin biosynthesis and insulin release of cryopreserved human fetal pancreas. Diabetes 31:238–241.
34. Kemp JA, Hurt SN, Brown J, et al (1981) Recovery and function of human fetal pancreas frozen to − 196 °C. Transplantation 32:10–15.
35. Tuch BE, Ng ABP, Jones A, et al (1984) Histologic differentiation of human fetal pancreatic explants transplanted into nude mice. Diabetes 33:1180–1187.
36. Paik S-G, Fleischer N, Shin S-I (1980) Insulin-dependent diabetes mellitus induced by subdiabetogenic doses of streptozotocin: Obligatory role of cell-mediated autoimmune processes. Proc Natl Acad Sci USA 77:6129–6133.
37. Buschard K, Rygaard J (1976) Restitution of streptozotocin induced diabetes mellitus in nude mice with pancreatic grafts from the rat. Acta Pathol Microbiol Scand (C) 84:221–226.
38. Tuch BE, Grigoriou S, Turtle JR (1986) Growth and hormonal content of human fetal pancreas passaged in athymic mice. Diabetes 35:464–469.
39. Povlson CO, Skakkeback NE, Rygaard J, et al (1974) Heterotransplantation of human foetal organs to the mouse mutant nude. Nature 248:247–249.
40. Usadel KH, Schwedes U, Bastert G, et al (1980) Transplantation of human fetal pancreas: Experience in thymus aplastic mice and rats and in a diabetic patient. Diabetes 29 [Suppl 1]:74–79.
41. Mandel TE, Georgiou HM (1983) Insulin secretion by fetal human pancreatic islets of Langerhans in prolonged organ culture. Diabetes 32:915–920.
42. Tuch BE, Jones A, Turtle JR (1985) Maturation of the response of human fetal pancreatic explants to glucose. Diabetologia 28:28–31.
43. Noonan RA, Walthall BJ, Godfrey WL, et al (1986) Reversal of diabetes in nude mice by xenograft transplant of cultured fetal pancreas. Diabetes 35 [Suppl 1]:138A.
44. Junod A, Lambert AE, Stauffacher W, et al (1969) Diabetogentic action of streptozotocin: Relationship of dose to metabolic response. J Clin Invest 48:2129–2139.
45. Groth, C-G, Andersson A, Bjorken C, et al (1980) Transplantation of fetal pancreatic microfragments via the portal vein to a diabetic patient. Diabetes 29 [Suppl 1]:80–83.
46. Tuch BE, Doran TJ, Messel N, et al (1985) Typing of human fetal organs for the histocompatibility antigens A, B and DR. Pathology 17:57–61.
47. Tuch BE, Sheil ARG, Ng ABP, et al (1986) Long term survival of human fetal pancreatic tissue transplanted into an insulin dependent diabetic patient. Diabet Med 3:24–28.
48. Tuch BE (1988) From nude mouse to man. In: Peterson CM, Jovanovic L, Formby B (eds) Human Fetal Islet Transplantation. Springer Verlag, New York (in press).

49. Freinkel N, Metzger BE (1979) Pregnancy as a tissue culture experience: the critical implications of maternal metabolism for fetal development. In Pregnancy Metabolism Diabetes and the Fetus. CIBA Foundation Symposium No 63, Excerpta Medica, Amsterdam, pp 3–23.

Part III Optimal Management

4
Oral Hypoglycemic Agents in the Treatment of Gestational Diabetes

EDWARD J. COETZEE AND W.P.U. JACKSON

Introduction

The use of oral antidiabetic agents in pregnancy is a most controversial topic. Many obstetricians and diabetologists vehemently oppose their use. Their reasons, however, are usually anecdotal or based on publications about oral agents that are no longer used in pregnancy. Yet, apart from the convenience to patients, which results in greater compliance, there are other reasons that suggest their use to be logical in women with non-insulin-dependent diabetes (NIDD). Such patients do not have a lack of insulin; they frequently have an excess of insulin production but, because of "insulin resistance," the hormone's message is imperfectly transmitted. Thus, use of drugs that alter this situation would be more logical than adding further insulin to a system that already has enough. There is evidence (which will be discussed later) that sulfonylureas and metformin do indeed influence events concerning carbohydrate metabolism at the cellular level. However, this does not negate the importance of diet, which we believe is the cornerstone of therapy for NIDD or gestational diabetes mellitus (GDM) (1).

Jorgen Pedersen (2) stated that he did not favor the use of either insulin or oral compounds in pregnant patients whose blood glucose levels could be sufficiently decreased with a restricted diet; we fully concur. At the same symposium Freinkel stated that although he respected and admired the groups that had presented their experience with oral antidiabetic agents, he would be remiss if he did not publicly voice his profound reservations about their use in pregnancy (3). We have the greatest respect for his concern, but we have no doubt that there is a place for the use of these drugs in GDM and in early NIDD. We hope to convince at least some doubters by the end of this chapter.

Definitions

Before proceeding, we must define gestational diabetes mellitus. The old definition of GDM was linked to a term no longer in vogue, namely, latent diabetes (4), which described a state characterized by normal glucose tolerance and reversible chemical or clinical diabetes in times of stress. Pregnancy was considered a particular stress, leading to GDM (5), which reverted to normal glucose tolerance after completion of the pregnancy. This definition has been superceded by that of the National Diabetes Data Group (NDDG) of the National Institutes of Health (6). It defines GDM as follows:

[A type of diabetes occurring in] pregnant women in whom the onset or recognition of diabetes or IGT (impaired glucose tolerance) occurs during pregnancy. Thus, diabetic women who become pregnant are not included in this class. In addition, after pregnancy terminates, the woman must be reclassified, either into diabetes mellitus or IGT, if her postpartum PG (plasma glucose) levels meet the criteria for those classes, or into previous abnormality of glucose tolerance (PrevAGT). In the majority of gestational diabetic women, glucose tolerance returns to normal postpartum, and the subject can be reclassified as PrevAGT. GDM is recommended as a separate class because of the special clinical features of the diabetes developing in pregnancy. Patients with asymptomatic, newly diagnosed diabetes in pregnancy, in whom there is no prior adverse obstetric history and in whom good control can be maintained with diet alone, are still at increased risk for perinatal morbidity and mortality. There is also an increased frequency of viable fetal loss.

This definition is practical and renders classification of patients easier. We have previously discussed the management of GDM (7), but as our publication appeared prior to the NDDG Report we used the unwieldy phrase: Diabetes "Newly diagnosed in pregnancy."

Essex et al (8) also had a problem with definition and proposed a simple classification that includes a single category of women in whom diabetes is diagnosed during pregnancy, regardless of whether the diabetes remits thereafter or not.

A common mistake is to use the term "gestational diabetes" as synonymous with class A diabetes (White's classification). Gabbe et al (9) wrote: "These women have also been designated class A diabetics by White (1949). They have a normal fasting serum glucose and an abnormal glucose tolerance test and require little dietary regulation." In fact, in 1949 White (10) stated that their evaluation was based on the prepregnancy state. Gestational diabetes was therefore *excluded*. Although White did modify her classification several times to allow the inclusion of gestational diabetes, in her final word in 1980 she upheld her first decision. Hare and White (11) decided that the White classification was intended to be used primarily for women who had established diabetes antedating pregnancy and that gestational diabetes should be considered separatedly whether insulin treated or not.

Another common error is to include only pregnant women with a normal fasting blood glucose (FBG) level (9,12). However, women with abnormal FBG levels may remit, and their glucose tolerance may return to normal after delivery, thus fulfilling the original definition of gestational diabetes.

Biochemical Criteria for Gestational Diabetes

The next thorny issue in the new definition is to decide the biochemical criteria for the terms "diabetes" and "impaired glucose tolerance." Having defined these concepts on the basis of tolerance to a 75-g oral glucose load in the nonpregnant state, the NDDG elected to define an abnormal glucose test in pregnancy according to the criteria of O'Sullivan and Mahan, which are based on a 100-g glucose load (13). Their criteria require that two or more of the following plasma glucose concentrations be met or exceeded: fasting, 105 mg/dL (5.8 mmol/L); 1 hour, 190 mg/dL (10.6 mmol/L); 2 hours, 165 mg/dL (9.2 mmol/L); 3 hours, 145 mg/dL (8.1 mmol/L).

The new definition of gestational diabetes and the criteria of O'Sullivan and Mahan were accepted by both the first and second workshop-conferences on gestational diabetes held in Chicago in 1979 (14) and in 1984 (15). However, in centers where other criteria have been established in different population groups, or with the use of glucose loads other than 100 g, their own local criteria should be continued (14,15). The International Congress on GDM clearly stated that other criteria in different population groups using different glucose levels are acceptable. Therefore, for this reason (i.e., that it is acceptable) our definition of gestational diabetes continues to be based on a 50-g oral glucose load, an amount of glucose chosen because during an epidemiologic study of diabetes in the various racial groups in Cape Town (16), it was found that the use of a 100-g glucose load resulted in an impossibly high prevalence of abnormal glucose tolerance. Thus, using a 50-g load and two standard deviations from the mean, venous plasma and an autoanalyzer glucose oxidase technique, we consider normal the following cutoff values:

Fasting, 100 mg/dL (5.5 mmol/L)
Peak, 180 mg/dL (10 mmol/L)
120 minutes, 126 mg/dL (7.0 mmol/L)

At least two abnormal values define an abnormal glucose tolerance test (GTT), and a diagnosis of gestational diabetes requires two abnormal glucose tolerance tests.

The Significance of Gestational Diabetes

Survey of the Literature

Has gestational diabetes any effect on the health of the mother and fetus? Is it important to make the diagnosis and will treatment change the outcome? The NDDG considered that GDM should be recognized as a separate entity because patients with asymptomatic, newly diagnosed diabetes in pregnancy, in whom there is no prior adverse obstetric history, are still at increased risk of perinatal mortality and morbidity even when good control can be maintained with diet alone. Furthermore, the NDDG believes that effective therapy could prevent much of the associated perinatal morbidity and mortality and that women with GDM have a high risk of developing diabetes 5 to 10 years later. This has the implied connotation that there might be some advice or therapy available, or still to be discovered, that might prevent this happening. The World Health Organization technical report was less certain (17). However, a prospective study revealed that the pregnancy-related risks were higher in women with GDM than in randomly selected nondiabetic women, even in centers providing good prenatal care (18). Perinatal mortality was 90 per 1,000 in GDM patients and 11 per 1,000 in patients with normal GTT, 25 years or older. In contrast to these results, Gabbe, in an oft-quoted publication (9), reported a low perinatal mortality (19 per 1,000) in women with GDM. As already pointed out, Gabbe's group represented a subsection of gestational diabetic women who had normal fasting plasma glucose levels and needed only mild dietary regulation. In fact, even in his study a subgroup of women who had a history of stillbirths had a perinatal mortality (PNM) of 88 per 1,000. Stallone and Ziel (19) also confused class A diabetes with GDM and put GDM patients who needed insulin into class B, calculating the incidence of PNM in patients who needed only mild dietary regulation. They concluded therefore that the PNM for GDM was 10 per 1,000, although in the seven patients who needed insulin the PNM was 430 per 1,000. The true overall PNM in their 107 patients was therefore 37/1,000.

Untreated Gestational Diabetes (Cape Town Experience)

We have been in the unique position to study a group of patients who had no treatment for their GDM (NDDG definition). The University of Cape Town Teaching Hospital, Groote Schuur, serves mainly an indigent, low socioeconomic population and its obstetric service delivers approximately 26,000 mothers annually. The clinics are often overcrowded and although we have a set of screening criteria (20) indicating when patients should have a GTT, some patients slip through the net, book late or not at all, and often miss clinic appointments or appointments for GTT. Thus, over a period of 10 years *53* patients who fulfilled our biochemical criteria for GDM received less than ten days of treatment for their GDM or absconded after initial treatment only to reappear at delivery (21). There were 13 stillbirths and one neonatal death, giving a PNM of 264 per 1,000. The PNM in the whole obstetric service during the same period was 30.8 per 1,000 while that in treated GDM patients was 14 per 1,000.

The treated and untreated groups had similar ethnic, age, and obesity distribution and the same obstetric care. In fact, 46 of the 53 "untreated" patients booked for obstetric care at a mean gestational age of 23 weeks, which is the usual time for all obstetric patients in our service. Even our unbooked nondiabetic patients did much better than our untreated GDM patients. In a study of 128 unbooked nondiabetic patients who received no obstetric care other than during labor, the PNM was 94 per 1,000, and five out of seven stillbirths were due to abruptio placentae. No stillbirth among the untreated GDM was due to abruptio placentae. Perinatal morbidity in this group was higher than that in the overall obstetric population. In particular, the prevalence of neonatal hypoglycemia and jaundice was double, and 37.5% of live-born infants weighed more than 3,899 g, compared with 6.5% of infants in the overall population. We can only conclude that in our population, GDM as defined by the NDGG has a profound influence on PNM and perinatal morbidity.

Treatment of Gestational Diabetes

In an editorial (22) in the *British Medical Journal* the question was asked: "If the risk of perinatal mortality is higher in cases of gestational diabetes, can anything be done to lower it?"

O'Sullivan (23) was one of the first clinicians to actively treat mild abnormal glucose tolerance when first diagnosed in pregnancy. In a study consisting of treated (10 units of insulin per day) patients, positive controls (no insulin), and negative controls (nondiabetic women), he could not demonstrate any difference in PNM between the treated and positive control patients, except for a reduction in the prevalence of large infants. In 1971 he reexamined the same patient cohort, now knowing which patients had become overtly diabetic in the interim (24). He defined these women as having been prediabetic at the time of the initial study and found a higher PNM at the time of the initial pregnancy among the offspring of the women who had not been treated than among the offspring of those who had.

Tyson and Hock (25) put the management of GDM on a more scientific basis when they declared that the objective of management in the pregnant diabetic patient (both gestational and pregestational) is to achieve physiologic glucose homeostasis through the use of diet and insulin. In their experience, maintenance of the plasma glucose concentration below 100 mg/dL (5.5 mmol/L), regardless of the severity of the diabetes, all but removes the risk of maternal-fetal complications due to diabetes. We fully agree with this statement, but we would like to add oral hypoglycemic agents to the above armamentarium.

History of the Oral Antidiabetic Agents

Sulfonylureas

The hypoglycemic action of these drugs was a serendipitous discovery made toward the end of World War II. While testing a sulfonylurea designated 2,254 R.P. for the possible treatment of typhoid fever, Janbon observed that many of his patients developed hypoglycemia. Loubatieres confirmed that the drug also caused hypoglycemia in dogs, provided that the pancreas was present (26).

MECHANISM OF ACTION

Despite three decades of use, the mode of action of sulfonylureas is still unclear. As they require the presence of functioning pancreatic tissue, it is obvious that they must have an effect on or via the pancreas. When given in single doses, they cause a prompt increase in the release of pre-formed insulin (27). However, both basal and stimulated insulin release return to pretreatment values weeks to months after therapy has been commenced, even when the improvement in glucose tolerance persists (28). The available circulating insulin therefore seems to be more effective, suggesting that the sulfonylureas may improve insulin-stimulated peripheral glucose disposal through a postreceptor action in muscle, liver, and adipocytes (29). An additional extrapancreatic action may be a reduction of hepatic glucose production through a still unknown mechanism (30).

Biguanides

While studying the effects of parathyroidectomy, it was discovered, once again quite unexpectedly, that guanidine derivatives had a hypoglycemic action (31). However, guanidine was too toxic to warrant therapeutic trials. Diguanidines (two guanidine molecules separated by a methylene chain) were next studied in diabetes. Synthalin A and B were selected for clinical use. Once again they proved too toxic. Eventually the biguanides (two guanidine molecules linked together by the elimination of one molecule of ammonia) were developed and widely used in diabetes. Although three biguanides, i.e., phenformin, buformin, and metformin, were used initially, phenformin has been discontinued because of a high risk of lactic acidosis (32,33). Metformin has rarely been implicated in lactic acidosis or other serious side effects (34) and is still widely used.

MECHANISM OF ACTION

Biguanides do not directly or indirectly stimulate the β-cells to secrete insulin. The site of action is therefore presumably extra-pancreatic. Some of the mechanisms for normalizing blood glucose levels that have been suggested are appetite suppression, decreased absorption of carbohydrate from the gastrointestinal tract (35), inhibition of hepatic gluconeogenesis (36), and enhancement of the peripheral action of insulin (37).

Use of the Sulfonylureas in Pregnancy: Survey of the Literature

Established Diabetes

In 1961 Endean and Smith (38) thought that the treatment of diabetes with oral agents had been a tremendous step forward and advocated its use in selected pregnant diabetic women. They then described three pregnancies in two mothers who had diabetic symptoms and a severe abnormality of the GTT who had been treated with tolbutamide throughout their pregnancies, and had three normal live infants of normal size. Jackson et al started a storm with their report of 42 women who had received tolbutamide or chlorpropamide during the whole or most of their pregnancy (39). The results were analyzed retrospectively from the clinical records, and the quality of blood glucose control was difficult to judge, especially because some of the patients had remained unsupervised for long periods. The majority of patients were Natal Indians living in Durban and "Cape Colored" living in Cape Town. The PNM rate in the sulfonylurea-treated group was approximately 50% whereas in 60 pregnant patients treated with insulin it was 20%. However, in the few (17) women treated with tolbutamide, the PNM was 23% (similar to that of the insulin-treated group). Among patients classified as being in poor control, the PNM was higher in the sulfonylureas than in the insulin-treated group (55% and 31%, respectively). Most patients received 500 mg of chlorpropamide daily, and in three patients who received only 250 mg of chlorpropamide daily, there was no PNM. Jackson et al concluded that chlorpropamide in a dosage of 500 mg daily appeared to be associated with a high PNM, although it might be safer at a lower dosage, and that tolbutamide appeared to be safe. The increased PNM was not due to congenital abnormalities. We now believe that the reason for the abysmal results obtained with the higher dose of chlorpropamide was poor diabetic control. At the same meeting, Dolger et al (40) reported 52 cases treated with tolbutamide, with a PNM of only 7.7% and only one significant congenital abnormality.

An interesting trial was also described by Miller et al (41). Among 42 pregnant patients, 25 acted as controls and did not receive tolbutamide.

Seven diabetic, six prediabetic, and four nondiabetic women received tolbutamide. The 17 treated patients received the last dose of tolbutamide 30 minutes to 15 hours prior to delivery. Tolbutamide blood levels were measured in maternal and placental blood and in the neonatal blood three hours after delivery. Tolbutamide was found in placental venous blood in higher concentrations than in maternal blood, and, surprisingly, the highest levels were found in the neonatal blood taken three hours after delivery. It was suggested that tolbutamide crosses the placental barrier and is not metabolized by the fetus. Blood glucose levels were measured in the cord blood and in the neonate 1, 2, and 3 hours after birth. Miller et al concluded:

The average blood sugar values obtained in the infants born to the diabetic mothers are also very similar to those studied by others. The main difference, however, is that our non-diabetic and diabetic mothers received tolbutamide. This would suggest that tolbutamide has little, if any, effect on the blood sugar in newborn infants born to patients treated with tolbutamide.

It is a great pity that the insulin levels were not measured in the cord blood and in the newborn of nondiabetic controls, as it is unlikely that such an experiment could ever be repeated today. Such data would have answered the question whether tolbutamide or any other sulfonylurea can directly stimulate insulin release from the pancreatic β-cells of the fetus and newborn.

The next significant contribution to the subject came from The Rare Disease Subcommittee of the Medical and Scientific Section, British Diabetic Association (42). They reported on 23 women treated with sulfonylurea drugs throughout the first and second trimester (15 women took chlorpropamide and eight women, tolbutamide). All but one had been taking the same drug at the time of conception. Unfortunately, we are not told what these patients were taking during the third trimester. An additional 18 women were treated with sulfonylurea drugs during the last trimester only (11 were on chlorpropamide, five on acetohexamide, and two on tolbutamide). The PNM in the first group was excellent—one stillbirth out of 23 (4.3%). In the second group it was poor, with six perinatal deaths (five stillbirths) out of 18 pregnancies (33%). Apart from one accessory auricle, there were no fetal deformities reported. The subcommittee regarded the number of casees too small to permit conclusions but made the following tentative comments:

There is no evidence of a teratogenic effect of sulphonylurea drugs usually employed in the human subject. There is as yet insufficient evidence to show whether these drugs have a harmful effect in the later stages of pregnancy. The apparent difference in the outcome of pregnancies in group A from those in group B cannot be explained because the numbers are small. It does perhaps accord with the observations of Pedersen and Brandstrup that women reporting early in pregnancy have a lower fetal loss rate than those who come late, for all but 3 of the women in group B had no treatment in the first six months of their pregnancy.

The difficulties involved with the use of insulin to control and manage diabetic mothers in an underdeveloped community have been pointed out by Douglas and Richards (43). Where no treatment was available, the PNM was 636 per 1,000, but in 34 chlorpropamide-treated patients the PNM was 118 per 1,000 in comparison with 42 patients treated with insulin who had a PNM of 167 per 1,000.

Two French investigators conducted a nationwide investigation into the use of oral hypoglycemic agents in pregnancy and recorded 90 such pregnancies (44). The PNM was 145 per 1,000 compared with a PNM of 157 and 190 per 1,000 in groups of pregnant diabetics treated with insulin during a similar period. From the literature they were able to analyze the results of 243 children born after administration of oral hypoglycemic drugs. Only three children had malformations, a frequency of 1.2%.

Notelowitz (45) reported on 104 pregnant diabetic women treated with sulfonylureas (58 with chlorpropamide and 46 with tolbutamide). The PNM was 137 per 1,000 in the chlorpropamide-treated mothers, 152 per 1,000 in the tolbutamide-treated mothers, and 170 per 1,000 in the insulin-treated mothers. There were only two cases of congenital abnormalities in the series, one of which occurred in the infant of a mother who had received tolbutamide. There were no cases of symptomatic neonatal hypoglycemia. The maximum dose of chlorpropamide used was 250 mg daily and that of tolbutamide 1.5 g.

Although the PNM of these early studies seem high compared with that achieved today, one must obviously assess them in the light of results achieved with insulin therapy over the same period.

Gestational Diabetes

These reports have dealt mainly with overtly insulin-dependent diabetic women, but they illustrate that when tolbutamide and chlorpropamide were used in appropriate doses, PNM and perinatal morbidity were not significantly different from those seen in insulin-treated patients. No single study has shown an increase in congenital abnormalities. Thus, these drugs should be safe for gestational diabetes as well. Sutherland and co-workers administered (46) 100 mg of chlorpropamide daily during pregnancy to 50 women with chemical diabetes that appeared for the first time during pregnancy and that was diagnosed by means of an intravenous GTT (increment index 2.97 or less). Seven consecutive patients were treated daily for an average of 11 weeks and then retested (with an intravenous GTT) 3 weeks after stopping the chlorpropamide. An improvement of carbohydrate tolerance was suggested as the mean increment index rose from 2.52 to 3.81, a significant difference ($p<.005$), assuming zero difference in patients not treated with chlorpropamide.

Sutherland et al also studied the birth weight and blood glucose kinetics of the neonate and measured insulin levels in cord blood; they concluded—

after suitable corrections for sex, gestational age, parity, social group, maternal height, and weight for height—that chlorpropamide therapy had not caused an excessive fetal weight gain. Nor had chlorpropamide treatment resulted in hyperinsulinism or exacerbated the usual neonatal hypoglycemia. Lastly, an intravenous glucose challenge was given to the newborn. The rate of glucose disposal was greater in the infants of chlorpropamide-treated mothers, but the insulin peak was lower. The PNM among the infants of chlorpropamide-treated mothers was higher than that of the untreated group (40 per 1,000 and 8 per 1,000, respectively). However, it is unlikely that either of the two neonatal deaths was attributable to chlorpropamide. The first death was due to the preterm delivery (32 weeks gestational age) e) of an infant who was thought to be growth retarded. The other neonate had a large diaphragmatic hernia and did not survive surgical correction.

In 1974 Sutherland et al (47) reviewed the outcome of 19 pregnancies in which diabetic mothers had received at least 200 mg of chlorpropamide daily. All perinatal deaths were among the poorly controlled mothers whose blood glucose level was > 170 mg/dL. There were two stillbirths and one neonatal death. All infants from poorly controlled mothers showed clinical or biochemical abnormalities, whereas when maternal diabetes was well-controlled (blood glucose level < 130 mg/dL) half the infants showed no clinical or biochemical abnormalities. In three infants cord arterial and venous blood was obtained for insulin levels. In one infant the insulin level was almost normal, in the second it was distinctly raised, and in the third it was very high (30, 83, and 500 μU/mL, respectively). The infant with the highest level was macrosomic but did not develop hypoglycemia; the mother was poorly controlled. Other indices of metabolic status such as glucose kinetics suggested that the neonates generally were in a mild state of hyperinsulinemia, but the data do not allow for discriminating whether this was due to chlorpropamide or to poor maternal blood glucose control.

The authors conclude with a cautious statement:

So far as it was possible on a clinical rating to assess the relative effects of the two potential stimuli of fetal hyperinsulinism in this series, chlorpropamide appeared to have the lesser effect, because it seems from this study that the infant's condition is more closely related to the control of maternal diabetes than to the total dosage of chlorpropamide taken during the pregnancy.

This article received favorable comment in a *Lancet* editorial (48):

The Aberdeen findings provide strong evidence that chlorpropamide in pregnancy is harmless to the fetus or infant and that good control of maternal diabetes, however this is achieved, is the most important contribution towards a successful outcome. Chlorpropamide therapy is best confined to pregnancy in women with mild diabetes, in whom good control can be attained with small doses. Chlorpropamide in this context seems sensible and worthy of wider usage, provided it is combined with strict attention to other aspects of diabetic control and expert obstetric management.

With characteristic Aberdonian thoroughness, 59 (56%) of the 106 children of chlorpropamide-treated mothers were followed for several years (49). They were assessed for growth, neurologic and intellectual ability, and glucose tolerance and compared with children of chemical diabetic mothers who had not been treated with drugs and of mothers who had been treated with insulin. There were no statistically significant differences between the groups with regard to growth or neurologic assessment. There appeared to be a significant impairment in glucose tolerance of children of mothers treated with insulin, but not in the children of the chlorpropamide-treated mothers, although among the latter, one developed insulin-dependent diabetes and two others have chemical diabetes.

Neonatal Hypoglycemia

In 1968 Zucker and Simon (50) reported the occurrence of prolonged symptomatic hypoglycemia in the neonate of a woman who had taken 500 mg of chlorpropamide daily and had received 250 mg of chlorpropamide on the morning of her delivery. The newborn did not respond to intravenous glucose or to glucagon administration and had to undergo exchange transfusion to remove the chlorpropamide from its blood. We believe that in this case, the clinicians had transgressed published guidelines concerning the use of chlorpropamide in pregnancy (51), namely that (a) chlorpropamide be used only under close supervision, (b) the dosage be limited to 250 mg daily, and (c) the drug be stopped about 10 days before delivery and insulin be substituted if necessary.

Four additional cases of severe neonatal hypoglycemia that did not respond to intravenous glucose, glucagon, and cortisone (singly or in combination) were reported by Kemball et al (52). Two of the neonates had to be treated with exchange transfusions to remove the hypoglycemic drug. One of the four patients was the infant of a woman who had received 1,000 mg daily doses of acetohexamide, which is on the high side for this preparation. Two other infants suffered fetal distress and asphyxia neonatorum; one of these had multiple congenital abnormalities and the other suffered a traumatic delivery. All four infants weighed more than 4,000 g and had the typical appearance of infants of poorly controlled diabetic mothers.

Biguanides in Pregnancy

Little has been written about biguanides in pregnancy. Sterne and Lavieuville (44) reported on 40 cases (32 on metformin and eight on phenformin), but most of their patients had been treated also with insulin. The

PNM was comparable to that prevailing at the time among insulin-treated patients, i.e., 15%.

The next reference to biguanides in pregnancy in the English-speaking literature was by Notelowitz (53), who used biguanides on the assumption that they would enhance the effectiveness of insulin and therefore correct the resistance to insulin observed in pregnancy. Although he published no details, the author stated that there were no untoward effects.

Stowers and Sutherland (54) used biguanides only in obese, chemical diabetic women who had failed to achieve normal blood glucose levels with dietary treatment. Thus, their experience was limited to four patients treated with phenformin and five patients treated with metformin for a mean period of 40 days before delivery. All the infants survived, although one was born prematurely after 29 weeks of gestation.

Finally, Pedersen (12) published 30 cases treated with oral hypoglycemic agents in pregnancy. Fifteen were treated with tolbutamide and 15 with metformin. No specific data are given for the 15 patients on metformin except that they were obese and that there were no drug failures among them. The PNM for the whole group of 42 patients (30 patients on drugs and 12 patients with "secondary failure") was 48 per 1,000 and two infants (4.8%) had congenital abnormalities. These results did not differ from those obtained in patients with White's class A at that time.

The Cape Town Trial

In 1974 we were asked to assume responsibility for all pregnant diabetic patients in the university service, approximately 80 to 100 patients per year. Ninety percent of our patients were noninsulin-dependent, and in these NIDDM patients 62 percent were discovered during pregnancy. The majority of these patients had a low socioeconomic background, a poor education, lived under difficult conditions, and compliance, especially to insulin therapy, was very poor. In view of the exceedingly high rate of PNM in untreated gestational diabetes discussed earlier, we adopted a therapeutic regimen designed to achieve the best possible control of the blood glucose levels by means of diet with or without oral hypoglycemic drugs. We chose glibenclamide (glyburide) rather than tolbutamide or chlorpropamide because it is a short-acting and potent drug (55).

Methods

Gestational diabetes was diagnosed according to the criteria already described. All patients with newly discovered diabetes were admitted to a special prenatal ward and placed on a supervised diet. Obese patients (more than 20% overweight) received a diet of 4,200 kJ (1,000 kcal); all other patients received either a diet of 5,900 kJ (1,400 kcal) or 6,700 kJ (1,600 kcal), appropriate for diabetes (1).

Capillary blood samples were taken five times daily at 0600, 1100, 1400, 1800, and 2000h, and the plasma glucose levels were estimated using a Beckmann glucose analyzer. The management was considered satisfactory if the fasting level was below 5.5 mmol/L (100 mg/dL), and all postprandial levels were below 6.7 mmol/L (120 mg/dL).

If these goals could not be reached by diet, metformin or glibenclamide was administered (see Figure 4.1). If the patient was obese, metformin was given initially; if not, glibenclamide was the first choice. At first we used daily doses of 1.5 to 3 g metformin or 5 to 20 mg glibenclamide. When the 850 mg metformin tablets became available, we gave one tablet two or three times daily for a total daily dose of 1,750 to 2,550 mg. After evaluating the initial results, the maximum dose for glibenclamide was lowered to 10 mg daily and for metformin to 2,550 mg daily (although more than 1,750 mg were seldom used) (6,56,57).

Standard hepatic and renal function tests were performed on each patient before oral drugs were administered. Urine was tested regularly with Ketostix®, and blood ketone concentrations were estimated when the early morning Ketostix estimate was repeatedly 2+. The diet was adjusted according to the results. If either metformin or glibenclamide alone failed to control the diabetes adequately, the drugs were given in combination. When this failed, the patients were placed on insulin, using soluble (Actrapid) and intermediate-acting (Monotard) forms. When satisfactory con-

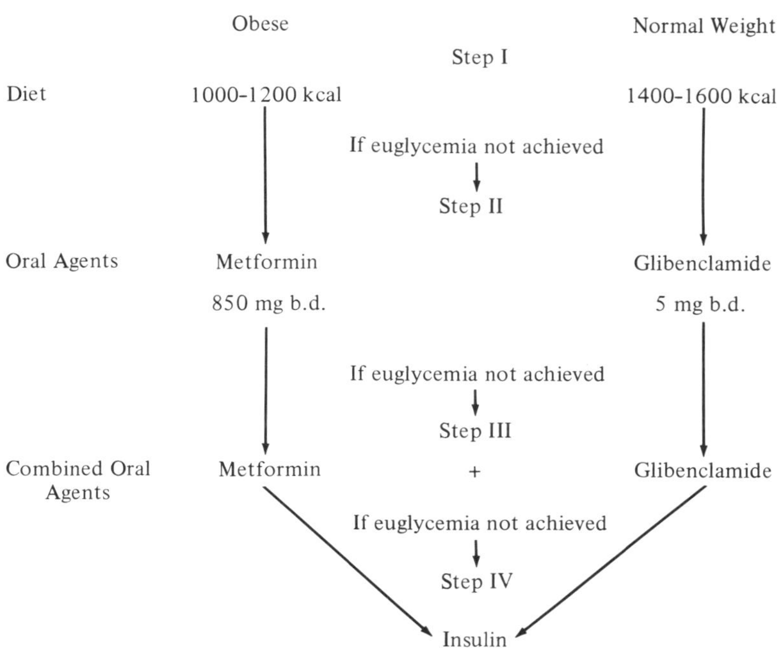

FIGURE 4.1. Treatment protocol for pregnant NIDD.

trol of the plasma glucose had been reached, the patient was discharged and followed in the outpatient clinic where frequent random estimations of blood glucose levels were made. If the degree of control worsened, the patient was readmitted to the ward.

All patients were readmitted after 32 weeks of gestation for strict control of the plasma glucose level, fetal monitoring (serial biparietal diameter by ultrasonography, fetal movements, and nonstressed cardiotopographs when indicated), placental lactogen, and bed rest.

When the results for 1977 were received (56), we found an unacceptable PNM for patients on combined metformin and glibenclamide therapy. The PNM appeared to be due largely to suboptimal blood glucose control, due in part to a refusal to accept insulin therapy when needed.

These results reinforced our resolve to achieve strict blood glucose control, and, after 1977, patients who did not do well on oral therapy alone received strong counsel to accept insulin injections for at least the remainder of their pregnancy. This policy appears to have been successful. Home monitoring techniques were not generally used because we felt that most of our patients would not be able to handle them.

Termination of Pregnancy

Because most of our patients booked late and could not recall their last menstrual period, amniocentesis was performed at 37+ weeks of gestation, estimated clinically or by ultrasound. Surfactant was detected by the foam test (58). If a foam score of at least 2+ was present, the pregnancy was terminated. When the foam score was 0 or 1+, the amniotic fluid phospholipid levels and, more recently, the presence or absence of phosphatidyl glycerol were assessed (59).

Labor was induced when a normal vaginal delivery was expected. Oral hypoglycemic agents were discontinued 14 hours before induction before 1978, but since then we have stopped the oral drugs approximately 36 hours before induction and have used continuous insulin infusion for the peripartum control of blood glucose levels. Thus, in the earliest part of the study, all diabetic women taking oral drugs or subcutaneous insulin were controlled with intermittent subcutaneous insulin during labor, but for the past 6 years these patients have received approximately 1 U of insulin subcutaneously or intravenously and 5 g dextrose intravenously per hour before and during labor. The rates of insulin and dextrose infusion have been adjusted independently according to the patient's glucose level and the presence of ketonuria. We attempted to maintain the blood glucose concentration between 5.0 and 7.2 mmol/L (90 and 130 mg/dL) as estimated by Dextrostix® strips. If delivery did not occur or was not imminent within 12 hours, the patient was delivered by cesarean section.

Neonates were transferred to a special care nursery for observation, usually for the first 24 hours after delivery. Dextrostix® readings were made hourly and hypoglycemia treated if necessary. Serum bilirubin was measured if the neonate appeared jaundiced.

Results

Between June 1974 and December 1983 we delivered 476 patients with gestational diabetes (57) but 53 did not receive any treatment for their GDM. Thirty-eight percent were 35 years or older and 70% were more than 20% overweight, according to the Kemsley tables (60). The PNM results are given in Table 4.1. Fifty-nine patients were given only metformin and 24 only glibenclamide; in addition, 43 patients received both drugs so that 102 patients received metformin and 67 received glibenclamide, alone or in combination, until delivery. In 39 additional patients, therapy with both drugs failed and treatment with insulin was begun before delivery (usually during the third trimester). The perinatal morbidity is shown in Table 4.2.

Less than 2% of the women suffered mild hypoglycemic effects from glibenclamide during pregnancy, none severe enough to require intravenous glucose. Two patients were unable to continue metformin because of gastrointestinal side effects. Lactic acidosis has not been seen. In addition, we have not observed a single case of serious neonatal hypoglycemia since we adopted the continuous insulin infusion regimen at term for all patients, whether they had been treated with insulin or with tablets.

Discussion

The pattern of diabetes in Cape Town may well reflect that of the developing world where NIDD in young people, often related to obesity, is becoming more prevalent. Such appears to be the case among Polynesian and Micronesian islanders (61,62), the Pima Indians (63), and possibly

TABLE 4.1. Therapy and outcome for pregnant women with gestational diabetes.

Therapy	No. of patients	SB	NND	PNM (per 1,000)
D	258	4	0	15
D + M	59	0	1	16
D + G	24	1	0	42
D + M + G	43	0	0	0
D + M + G → I	39	0	0	0
Total	423	5	1	14
"Untreated"	53	13	1	264

D = diet only, M = metformin, G = glibenclamide, I = insulin.
D + M + G → I = diet, metformin, and glibenclamide later transferred to insulin.
NND = neonatal death, PNM = perinatal mortality rate, SB = stillborn.

TABLE 4.2. Neonatal morbidity (in percentages) among women with gestational diabetes.

Therapy	LGA*	Low birth weight	Hypoglycemia	Jaundice	Congenital abnormalities[†]
Diet only	17	5	3	13	2
Metformin	16	19	6	25	8
Glibenclamide	22	0	17	9	0
D + M + G	14	7	14	47	9
D + M + G → I	18	13	8	33	10
Untreated	38	3	13	18	10

*Large for gestational age or high birth weight ≥ 3,900 g; low birthweight is < 2,500 g; hypoglycemia is < 25 mg/ dL or1.4 mmol/L; jaundice needs phototherapy.
[†]None of these patients were on oral agents in the first trimester.

other North American Indians (64). In these communities diabetes is often first discovered during pregnancy because of active screening programs. Another high-risk population for gestational diabetes is the expatriate Asian Indian community that has often adopted new dietary habits and socio-economic patterns. This has been clearly shown in South Africa (65), Trinidad (66), South East Asia, and Fiji (61).

From a survey of the literature it would seem that even old-fashioned sulfonylureas such as chlorpropamide and tolbutamide gave as good peri-natal results as insulin, providing certain doses are not exceeded. Fetal hypoglycemia could be a problem with chlorpropamide but there is no evidence of teratogenesis.

Our own studies confirm the notion that in NIDD women whose oral treatment started before the onset of pregnancy, the oral agents are not teratogenic (67). Furthermore, since the diagnosis of gestational diabetes is seldom made during the first trimester, an unfounded fear of terato-genesis should not influence the choice of medication.

On the basis of our results we believe that provided euglycemia is achieved, glibenclamide and metformin can be used in gestational diabetic women. Certain guidelines are, however, important. The maximum dosage for metformin should be 1,750 mg daily and maximum dose for gliben-clamide 10 mg daily. Both should be given in divided doses. From our work in established diabetic women (56,57) and from an ongoing study on amniotic fluid insulin levels in diabetic mothers, we think that even mild hyperglycemia can stimulate the mature fetal β-cells, increase their sensitivity to sulfonylureas and increase the risk of severe fetal hyper-insulinism. Thus, we hypothesize that if the fetal β-cell has not been ac-tivated by hyperglycemia, it is not responsive (or is less responsive) to sulfonylureas; therefore, we do not start treatment with sulfonylureas late in the third trimester unless we are sure that the maternal blood glucose levels have been reasonably normal.

The use of the short-acting glibenclamide has been a major breakthrough, but it is still preferable to allow a 24-hour "washout" period before delivery. During this time and throughout labor we attempt to achieve optimal blood glucose control using continuous insulin pumps. We have not had more than the most transient of hypoglycemia (never requiring treatment) on this regimen. Since we now tend to deliver our patients at a later gestational age than previously, several patients have gone into spontaneous labor while still on glibenclamide. Nevertheless, we have encountered no problems. Nor have we seen any evidence that a combination of metformin and anesthesia results in lactic acidosis in 56 patients who underwent cesarean section (68).

Conclusion

Only a large-scale randomized trial can decide whether insulin or the oral agents are safer for the fetus. We are now embarking on such a trial.

In the meantime, a PNM of 14 per 1,000 observed in our population of disadvantaged women with gestational diabetes suggests that a combined therapy with diet, metformin, and glibenclamide—and insulin as a last resort—may be cautiously recommended, for we believe that the secret of successful perinatal outcomes in all pregnant diabetic patients lies more in the achievement of excellent blood glucose levels than in the means of achieving it.

Editor's Note. Although the editor fully supports the above discussion, it must be noted that in the United States oral hypoglycemic agents are not approved for use during pregnancy. (L.J.)

References

1. Coetzee EJ, Jackson WPU (1985) Nutritional management of pregnant diabetic woman. In: Jovanovic L, Petersen CM (eds) Contemporary Issues in Clinical Nutrition 8. Nutrition and Diabetes. Alan R Liss Inc, New York, pp 121–132.
2. Pedersen J, Molsted-Pedersten L (1975) Oral "Anti-diabetic" compounds in Pregnancy. In: Camerini-Davalos RA, Cole HS (eds) Early Diabetes in Early Life. Academic Press, New York, San Francisco, London, pp 487–494.
3. Freinkel N (1975) Discussion. In: Camerini-Davalos RA, Cole HS (eds) Early Diabetes in Early Life. Academic Press, New York, San Francisco, London, pp 517–518.
4. Fitzgerald MG, Keen H (1964) Diagnostic Classification of Diabetes. Br Med J i:1568.
5. Brudenell M, Beard R (1972) Diabetes in Pregnancy. Clin Endocrinol Metab i:673–695.
6. National Diabetes Data Group (1979) Classification and diagnosis of diabetes mellitus and other categories of glucose intolerance. Diabetes 28:1039–1957.

7. Coetzee EJ, Jackson WPU (1979) Diabetes newly diagnosed during pregnancy. A 4-year study at Groote Schuur Hospital. S Afr Med J 56:467–475.
8. Essex NL, Pyke DA, Watkins PJ, Brudenell JM, Gamsu HR (1973) Diabetic Pregnancy. Br Med J 4:89–93.
9. Gabbe SG, Mestman JH, Freeman RK, Anderson GV, Lowensohn RI (1977) Management and outcome of Class A diabetes mellitus. Am J Obstet Gynecol 127:465–469.
10. White P (1949) Pregnancy complicating diabetes. Am J Med 7:609–616.
11. Hare JW, White P (1980) Gestational diabetes and the White Classification. Diabetes Care 3:194.
12. Pedersen J (1977) The pregnant diabetic and her newborn, ed 2. Munksgaard, Copenhagen, Williams & Wilkens, Baltimore, pp 22–45.
13. O'Sullivan JB, Mahan CM (1964) Criteria for the oral glucose tolerance test in pregnancy. Diabetes 13:278–285.
14. Workshop Chairman Report (Symposium on Gestational Diabetes) (1980) Summary and recommendations. Diabetes Care 3:499–501.
15. Summary and Recommendations of the Second International Workshop—Conference on Gestational Diabetes Mellitus (1985) Diabetes 34 [Suppl 2]:123–126.
16. Jackson WPU (1964) On diabetes mellitus. C C Thomas, Springfield, pp 129–142.
17. WHO Expert Committee on Diabetes Mellitus (1980). Technical Report Series (2nd Report), Geneva, p 646.
18. O'Sullivan JB, Charles D, Mahan CM, Dandrow RV (1973) Gestational diabetes and perinatal mortality rate. Am J Obstet Gynecol 116:901–904.
19. Stallone LA, Ziel HK (1974) Management of gestational diabetes. Am J Obstet Gynecol 119:1091–1094.
20. Jackson WPU, Coetzee EJ (1979) Glycosuria as an indication for glucose tolerance testing during pregnancy. S Afr Med J 56:921–923.
21. Coetzee EJ, Jackson WPU (1986) Perinatal mortality and morbidity in the untreated non-insulin-dependent diabetic. Abstracts from XVII meeting of the Diabetic Pregnancy Study Group of the European Association for the Study of Diabetes, p 28.
22. Editorial (1974) Gestational Diabetes. Br Med J (i): 167–168.
23. O'Sullivan JB, Gellis SS, Dandrow RV, Tenney BO (1966) The potential diabetic and her treatment in pregnancy. Obstet Gynecol 27:683–689.
24. O'Sullivan JB, Charles D, Dandrow RV (1971) Treatment of verified prediabetics in pregnancy. J Reprod Med 7:21–24.
25. Tyson JE, Hock RA (1976) Gestational and pregestational diabetes. An approach to therapy. Am J Obstet Gynecol 125:1009–1027.
26. Loubatieres A (1969) History and development of oral treatment of diabetes. In: Campbell GD (ed) Oral hypoglycaemic Agents. Pharamcology and Therapeutics. Academic Press, London, New York, pp 1–22.
27. Pfeifer MA, Halton JB, Judzewitsch RG, Beard JC, Best JD, Ward WK, Porte D (1984) Acute and chronic effects of sulphonylurea drugs in pancreatic islet function in man. Diabetes Care 7 [Suppl 1]:25–34.
28. Reaven G, Dray J (1967) Effects of chlorpropamide on serum glucose and immunoreactive insulin concentrations in patients with maturity onset diabetes mellitus. Diabetes 16:487–492.

29. Lebovitz HE (1984) Cellular loci of sulfonylurea actions. Diabetes Care 7 [Suppl 1]:67–71.
30. Defronzo RA, Simson DC (1984) Oral sulfonylurea. Agents suppress hepatic glucose production in non-insulin-dependent diabetic individuals. Diabetes Care 7 [Suppl 1]:72–80.
31. Sterne J (1969) Pharmacology and mode of action of the hypoglycaemic guanidine derivatives. In: Campbell GD (ed) Oral hypoglycaemic Agents. Pharmacology and Therapeutics. Academic Press, London, New York, pp 193–245.
32. Luft D, Schmulling RM, Eggstein M (1978) Lactic acidosis in biguanide-treated diabetics. A review of 330 cases. Diabetologia 14:75–87.
33. Vinik AI, Jackson WPU (1974) Lactic acidosis in diabetics. S Afr Med J 48:2021–2026.
34. Clarke BF, Campbell IW (1977) Comparison of metformin and chlorpropamide in non-obese, maturity-onset diabetics uncontrolled by diet. Br Med J 2:1576–1578.
35. Caspary WF, Creutzfelder W (1971) Analysis of the inhibitory effect of biguanides on glucose absorption. Inhibition of active sugar transport. Diabetologia 7:379–385.
36. Natrass M, Todd PG, Hinks L, Lloyd B, Alberti KGMM (1977) Comparative effects of phenformin, metformin and glibenclamide on metabolic rhythms in maturity-onset diabetics. Diabetologia 13:145–152.
37. Sterne J, Junien JL (1981) Metformin: Pharmacological mechanisms of the antidiabetic and antilipidic effects and clinical consequences. In: Van der Kuy A, Hulst SG (eds) Biguanide therapy today. Royal Society of Medicine: International Congress and Symposium Series No. 48. Royal Soc of Med, London, pp 3–13.
38. Endean DH, Smith GJ (1961) Use of tolbutamide in pregnant diabetics. J Michigan State Med Soc 60:1436–1438.
39. Jackson WPU, Campbell GD, Notelowitz M, Blumsohn D (1962) Tolbutamide and chlorpropamide during pregnancy in human diabetics. Diabetes 11 [Suppl]:98–101.
40. Dolger H, Bookman JJ, Nehemias C (1962) The diagnostic and therapeutic value of tolbutamide in pregnant diabetics. Diabetes 11 [Suppl]:97–98.
41. Miller DI, Wishinsky H, Thompson G (1962) Transfer to tolbutamide across the human placenta. Diabetes 11 [Suppl]:93–97.
42. Malins JM, Cooke AM, Pyke DA, Fitzgerald MG (1964) Sulfonylurea drugs in pregnancy (Letter). Br Med J ii:187.
43. Douglas CP, Richards R (1967) Use of chlorpropamide in the treatment of diabetes in pregnancy. Diabetes 16:60–61.
44. Sterne J, Lavieuville M (1968) Biguanides in pregnancy (Translated) Paper presented at symposium on the biguanides. Rimini, October 1968.
45. Notelowitz M (1971) Sulfonylurea therapy in the treatment of the pregnant diabetic. S Afr Med J 45:226–229.
46. Sutherland HW, Stowers JM, Cormack JD, Bewsher PD (1973) Evaluation of chlorpropamide in chemical diabetes diagnosed during pregnancy. Br Med J i:9–13.
47. Sutherland HW, Bewsher PD, Cormack JD, Hughes CRT, Reid A, Russell G, Stowers J (1974) Effect of moderate-dosage of chlorpropamide in pregnancy on fetal outcome. Arch Dis Child 49:283–291.

48. Chlorpropamide in diabetic pregnancy (1974) (Editorial) Lancet ii:32.
49. Reid JA, Russell G (1979) Qualitative assessment of children of known-gestational diabetic mothers. In: Sutherland HW, Stowers JM (eds) Carbohydrate Metabolism in Pregnancy and the Newborn. Springer-Verlag, Berlin, Heidelberg, New York, p 462–477.
50. Zucker P, Simon G (1968) Prolonged symptomatic neonatal hypoglycemia associated with maternal chlorpropamide therapy. Pediatrics 42:824–825.
51. Jackson WPU, Campbell GD (1963) Chlorpropamide and perinatal mortality (Letter) Br Med J ii:1652.
52. Kemball ML, McIver C, Milner RDG, Nourse CH, Schiff D, Tierman JR (1970) Neonatal hypoglycaemia in infants of diabetic mothers given sulfonylurea drugs in pregnancy. Arch Dis Child 45:696–701.
53. Notelowitz M (1974) Oral hypoglycaemic therapy in diabetic pregnancies. Lancet ii:902–903.
54. Stowers JM, Sutherland HW (1975) The use of sulfonylureas, biguanides and insulin in pregnancy. In: Sutherland HW, Stower JM (eds) Carbohydrate metabolism in pregnancy and the newborn. Churchill & Livingstone, Edinburgh, pp 205–220.
55. Balant L (1981) Clinical pharmacokinetics of sulfonylurea hypoglycaemic drugs. Clin Pharmacol, 6:215–241.
56. Coetzee EJ, Jackson WPU (1980) Pregnancy in established non-insulin-dependent diabetics. S Afr Med J 58:795–802.
57. Coetzee EJ, Jackson WPU (1986) The management t of non-insulin-dependent diabetes during pregnancy. Diabetes Res Clin Pract 1:281–287.
58. Gunston KD, Davey DA (1978) The bubble test as a measure of amniotic fluid surfactant and as a predictor of hyaline membrane disease. S Afr Med J 54:495–497.
59. Hallman M, Kulovich M, Kirkpatrick E, Sugarman RG, Gluck L (1976) Phosphatidylinositol and phosphatidylglycerol in amniotic fluid: Indices of lung maturity. Am J Obstet Gynecol 125:613–617.
60. Kemsley WFF (1952) Body weight at different ages and heights. Ann Eugenics (London) 16:316–334.
61. Ekoe JM (1986) Recent trends in prevalence and incidence of diabetes mellitus syndrome in the world. Diabetes Res Clin Pract, 1:249–264.
62. Zimmet P, Taft P, Guinea A, Guthrie W, Thomas K (1977) The high prevalence of diabetes mellitus on a Central Pacific Island. Diabetologia 13:111–115.
63. Bennett P, Burch TA, Miller M (1971) Diabetes mellitus in American (Pima) Indians. Lancet ii:125–128.
64. West KM (1974) Diabetes in American Indians and other Native populations of the New World. Diabetes 23:841–855.
65. Jackson WPU, Van Mieghem W, Marine N, Keller P, Edelstein I (1974) Diabetes among a Tamilian Indian Community in Cape Town. S Afr Med J 48:1839–1843.
66. Poon-King T, Henry MV, Rampersad F (1968) Prevalence and natural history of diabetes in Trinidad. Lancet i:155–160.
67. Coetzee EJ, Jackson WPU (1984) Oral hypoglycaemics in the first trimester and fetal outcome. S Afr Med J 65:635–537.
68. Jackson WPU, Coetzee EJ (1979) Side-effects of metformin (Letter) S Afr Med J 56:1113.

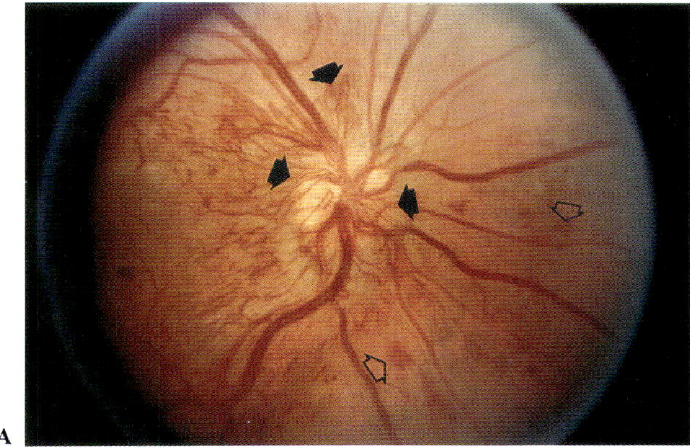

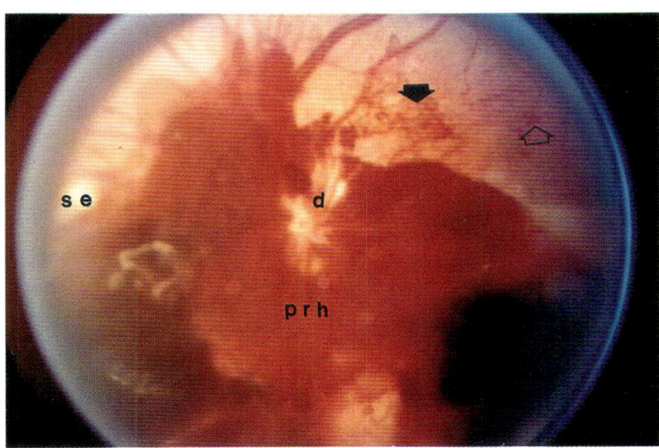

FIGURE 5.4. **A:** Fundus photograph of the right eye taken 2 weeks after delivery. There is exuberant new vessel formation on the optic disc (black arrows), and retinal hemorrhages (open arrows) are also seen. **B:** Fundus photograph of the left eye. The optic disc (d) is obscured by preretinal hemorrhage (prh). Fibrous proliferation, soft exudate (se), new vessels (solid arrow), and retinal hemorrhage (open arrow) can also be seen.

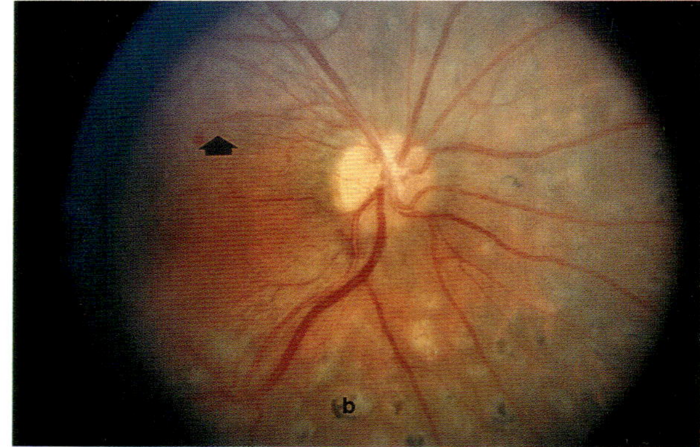

C

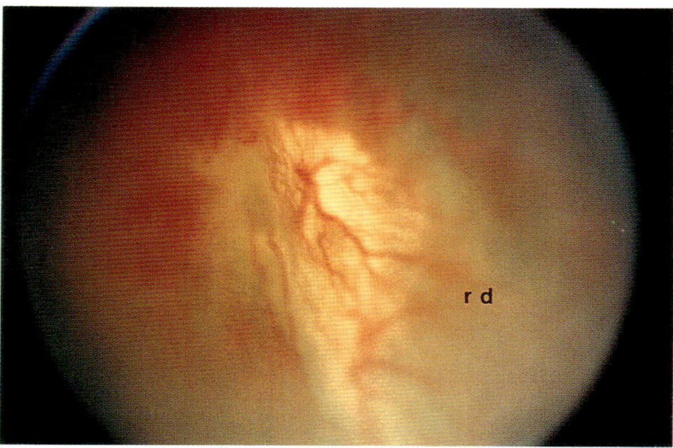

D

FIGURE 5.4. **C:** Photograph taken after completion of laser treatment. Pigmented and atrophic laser burns (b) are evident. Fibrous tissue overlies the optic disc and residual new vessels are seen (dark arrow). **D:** Photograph of the left eye taken at the same time as **C** was taken. There has been massive proliferation of fibrous tissue and there are residual new vessels that have caused a retinal detachment (rd).

5
Diabetic Retinopathy During Pregnancy

BARBARA E.K. KLEIN

Background

Before the development of a clinically useful form of insulin, the prognosis for insulin-dependent diabetes patients was grim. When a young woman with the condition became pregnant, she and her offspring rarely survived the pregnancy. With the development of insulin, short-term survival was more likely to occur. We then had the dubious privilege of observing the long-term complications and disabilities that accompany diabetes of long duration (1). The large number of diabetic individuals followed at the Joslin Clinic has been a source of much of the information concerning the problems encountered in pregnancy by these patients. White reported that 50% of all pregnant women followed at that institution between January 1936 and January 1965 had vascular lesions, and 10% of them had "malignant angiopathy." The rate of spontaneous abortions in these women was high, and the mothers often experienced severe hypoglycemic episodes during the pregnancy. Specifically, in 2,000 cases of obstetrical diabetes White found proliferative retinopathic changes in 87 cases. Of the 20 eyes that had sustained a hemorrhage, 11 progressed to blindness. Viable infants resulted from 74% of these cases (2). Cassar and colleagues reported that in 20% of 67 pregnant women with retinopathy, the lesions progressed during pregnancy (3). Similarly, Jervell et al reported a progression of retinopathy in 68 of 234 women who were followed through pregnancy at the Rikshospitalet in Oslo (4).

Clinical Cases

The problems of retinopathy in pregnancy have come to special attention because of the varied course of this complication. Some illustrative cases are described below.

Case 1

This patient had had insulin-dependent diabetes for nearly 12 years before she became pregnant for the first time. Figure 5.1A is a photograph of the optic disc taken during the first trimester of that pregnancy. Her visual acuity was 20/16. There was progression of the nonproliferative retinopathy during pregnancy (Figure 5.1B) but no proliferative changes developed, and the vision remained 20/16.

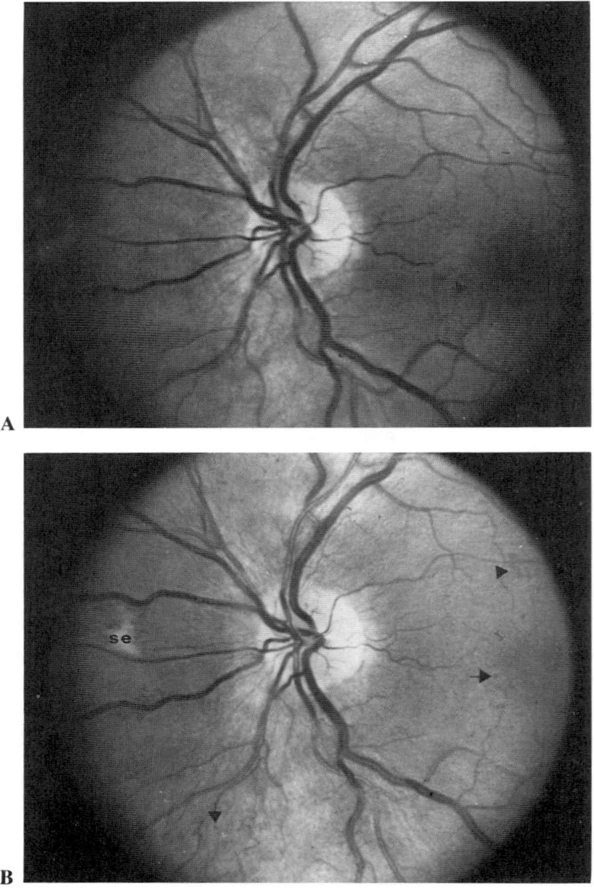

FIGURE 5.1. **A:** Fundus photograph of the left optic disc taken during the first trimester of pregnancy. The patient had a 12-year history of diabetes mellitus. A flame-shaped hemorrhage (arrow) is seen in the macular area. **B:** Fundus photograph of the left optic disc of the same patient taken during the postpartum period. Soft-exudate (se), intraretinal microvascular abnormalities (solid arrow head), and retinal microaneurysms are present (arrow). These lesions represent progression of nonproliferative retinopathy.

Case 2

This young woman was first seen nearly 2 years prior to her pregnancy. She, too, had had diabetes for about 12 years. Nonproliferative retinopathy was present (Figure 5.2A) but the visual acuity was 20/16. Two years later during the first trimester of her pregnancy more retinopathy was present and the vision had dropped to 20/25 (Figure 5.2B). She did not comply with the recommendation to return for close follow-up for the remainder of the first and for the second trimester. She did return during the third trimester. Her vision at that time was 5/200 and the fundus photos showed severe changes due to diabetic retinopathy (Figure 5.2C). At that time she was more receptive to suggestions for follow-up and was treated with laser photocoagulation. Figure 5.2D was taken after delivery and after completion of the photocoagulation treatment. Vision was 20/80 and there was regression of the proliferative retinopathy. There was mottling and dragging of the macula.

Case 3

This patient was first seen about 3 years before pregnancy. She had had diabetes for nearly 19 years at the time of these photographs (Figure 5.3A). Her vision was 20/16. She was seen a year later and was still not pregnant. The fundus and vision were virtually unchanged.

During the first trimester of pregnancy, moderate nonproliferative retinopathy with macular edema were present and the vision dropped to 20/40.

Figure 5.3B is a photograph taken during the third trimester when she was hospitalized for toxemia. Her vision was 5/200. Along with proliferative changes and macular edema, anterior segment rubeosis was present. Because of her severe toxemia at this time, her obstetricians were reluctant to allow any procedures before delivery. After delivery, fluorescein angiography was performed documenting marked ischemia (Figure 5.3C) of the fundus. At this point, aggressive photocoagulation was performed.

Figure 5.3D is a photograph taken during the postpartum period. Some proliferative changes persist, but the fundus is quieter. Her vision was 20/160. She has had no further laser treatment either for the fundus or for the anterior segment rubeosis.

Case 4

This patient was diagnosed as an insulin-dependent diabetic at 11 years of age. She was apparently asymptomatic with regard to ocular problems for the next 15 years. She was seen after that interval by an ophthalmologist during the course of her first pregnancy. The ophthalmologist described

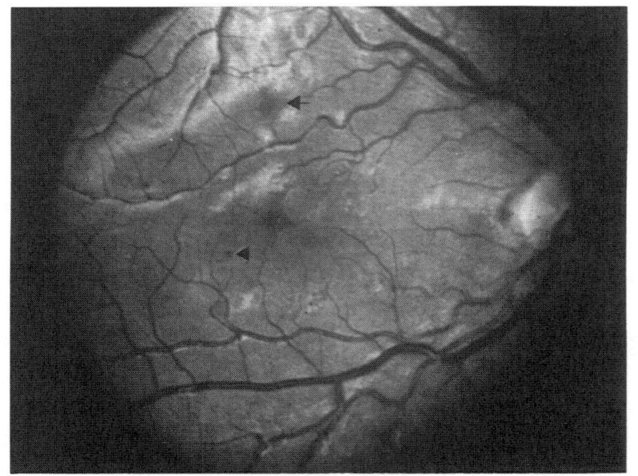

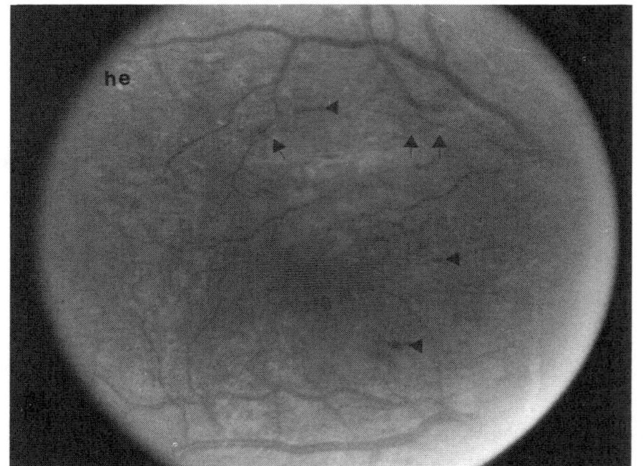
he

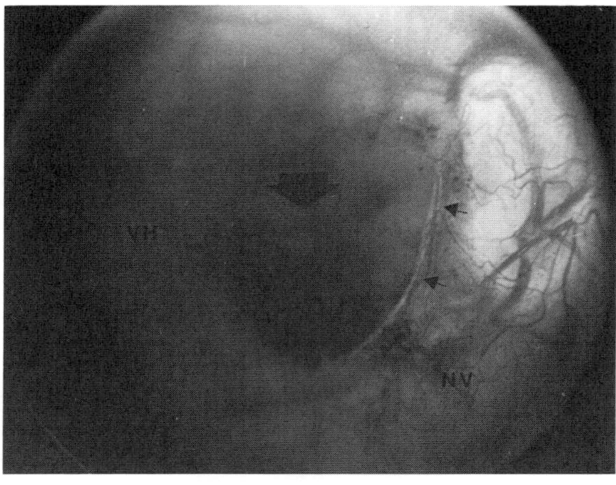
VH
NV

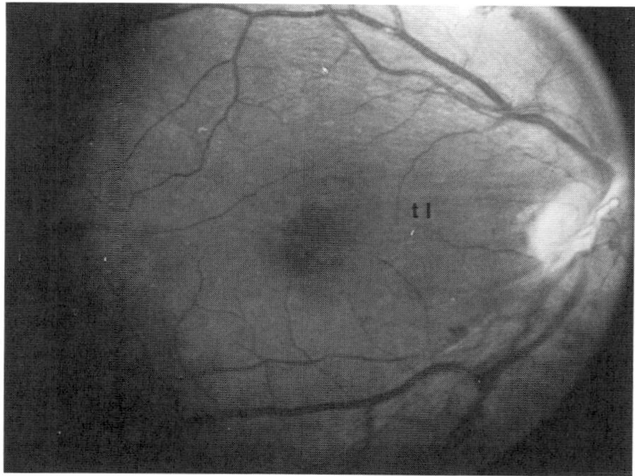

D

FIGURE 5.2. **A:** Fundus photograph of the macula of the right eye of case 2. The picture was taken two years before pregnancy. Nonproliferative retinopathy consisting of retinal hemorrhage (arrowhead) and intraretinal microvascular abnormalities (arrow) are present. **B:** Photograph of the macula of the same eye taken during the first trimester of pregnancy. There are more retinal hemorrhages (arrowheads) and intraretinal microvascular abnormalities (arrows) than in the previous photograph. In addition, hard exudate (he) can be seen. **C:** Photograph of the left eye of case 2 taken during the third trimester of pregnancy. Retinal hemorrhage, preretinal hemorrhage (large dark arrow), and vitreous hemorrhage (VH), which obscures part of the retina, are all present. New vessel formation (NV) and fibrous tissue (small arrows) are abundant. **D:** Photograph taken during the postpartum period. There are traction lines (tl) in the retina indicating dragging of macula. Fibrous tissue proliferation and some new vessels remain.

"minimal retinopathy." Two weeks after delivery she was seen at the University of Wisconsin Retina Clinic.

Photographs were taken of the optic disc of the right eye at the time of that visit (Figure 5.4A; see Plates 1 and 2 following page 76). The vision in this eye was 20/20. Extensive proliferative retinopathy on the optic disc was present.

The corresponding photograph of the left eye is seen in Figure 5.4B. The vision in this eye was 20/50. New vessels and hemorrhage were found. Panretinal photocoagulation in both eyes was performed in multiple sessions. The visual acuity decreased markedly in the left eye after treatment.

Figure 5.4C was taken after laser treatment. There has been regression of the neovascularization of the optic disc. The vision was 20/20. Figure 5.4D is a photograph of the left eye. The vision was sufficient to count fingers only. A vitrectomy was considered but the risks were thought to be too great. No further laser treatment was performed. One year later she was found to have vision of 20/20 in the right eye and only light perception in the left eye. In addition, she had developed rubeotic glaucoma

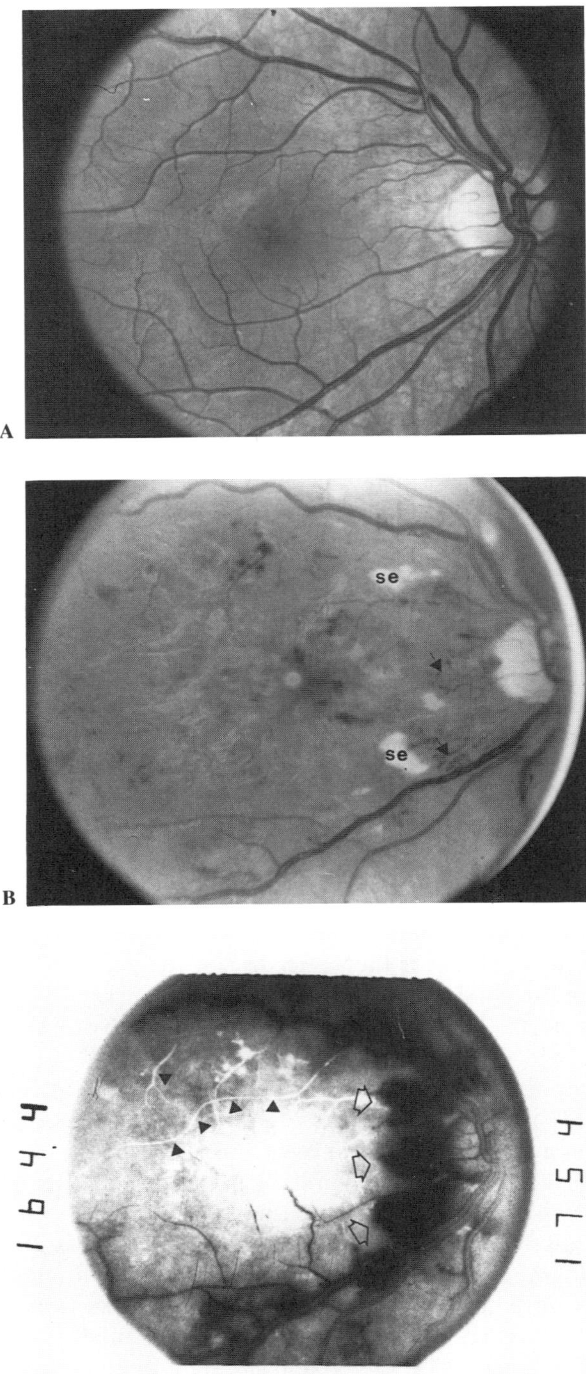

A
se
se
B
C

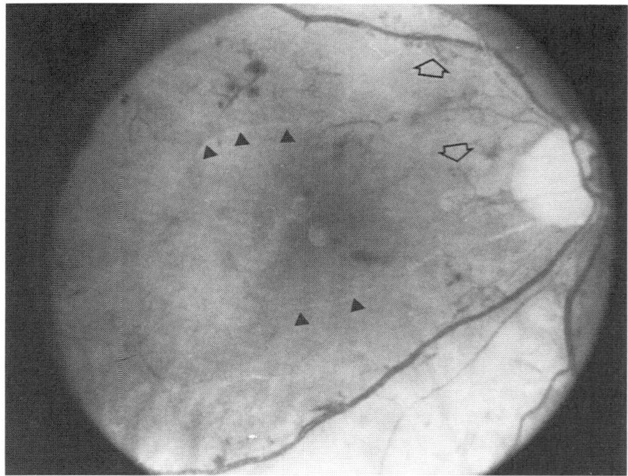

FIGURE 5.3. **A:** Photograph of the right eye. It shows early lesions of nonproliferative retinopathy consisting of retinal hemorrhages and microaneurysms. This is the appearance of the ocular fundus of case 3 before pregnancy. **B:** Photograph taken during third trimester of pregnancy. The patient was toxemic, and visual acuity was 5/200. There was marked progression of retinopathy. Retinal hemorrhage, intraretinal microvascular abnormalities, soft exudates (se), and new vessel formation (arrows) are all present. **C:** This is the negative of a photograph taken from a fluorescein angiogram series of the right eye. There are stringy, white, nonperfused blood vessels (solid arrowheads), with the macular area showing a large area of decreased perfusion (large whitish central area). Areas of abnormal leakage of the fluorescein dye (open arrows) can be seen. **D:** Photograph taken during the postpartum visit after extensive retinal photocoagulation treatment. Nonperfused vessels remain (solid arrowheads). There are residual new vessels present (open arrows).

in the left eye. One year following that visit, vision in the right eye was 20/30 and the retina appeared to be stable. There was no light perception at all in the left eye. At this time the patient decided that the pain in the left eye was severe enough to request enucleation. This was performed. The patient has had stable vision in her remaining right eye.

These case histories suggest that pregnancy may be a risk factor for the development and/or progression of diabetic retinopathy. However, to determine whether pregnancy is, in fact, an independent risk factor, one needs to be aware of the other factors that influence diabetic retinopathy.

Risk Factors for Retinopathy

The duration of diabetes is most closely associated with the presence of retinopathy, a finding reported in several studies (5–8) and confirmed recently by the Wisconsin Epidemiological Study of Diabetic Retinopathy

(WESDR) (9). In the WESDR, 17% of persons who had diabetes for fewer than 5 years and 97.5% of persons who had diabetes for 15 or more years had diabetic retinopathy. The effect of duration was noted in the insulin-taking younger onset patients as well as in the older onset patients (9,10). Not only the prevalence of retinopathy increases with the longer duration of diabetes, but the severity of retinopathy increases as well (9,10) (Figure 5.5).

The severity of retinopathy at the beginning of an observation period is thought to be significant in predicting subsequent changes in retinopathy. In another study done in Wisconsin, 191 persons with insulin-dependent diabetes who had had the disease for 5 years or more were followed for an additional 6 years. The rate of progression varied, depending on whether there was no retinopathy, minimal to mild retinopathy, or moderate retinopathy at the first examination (11). In the Diabetic Retinopathy Study, persons with severe nonproliferative retinopathy had a greater rate of progression than persons at other levels of severity (12). Part of the difficulty when using current severity to predict a time course for subsequent retinopathy is that although progression usually occurs according to a fairly predictable pattern, the scale of severity of retinopathy cannot be expressed in units of known size and the rate of progression varies. The usual pattern is for persons with no retinopathy to develop microaneurysms before developing other retinal vascular abnormalities, and microaneurysms tend to occur before new vessel formation, which precedes preretinal and vitreous hemorrhage. In the 172 patients followed by Horvat et al through pregnancy, the severity of retinopathy at the onset of preg-

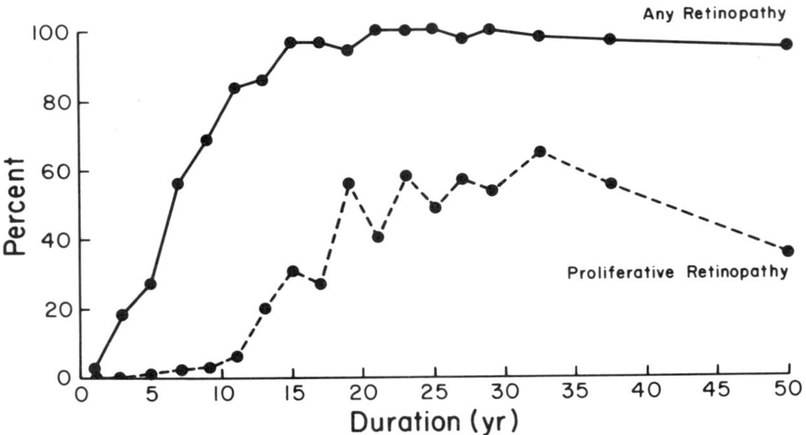

FIGURE 5.5. Frequency of retinopathy or proliferative retinopathy by duration of diabetes in years. (Reprinted with permission from Klein et al (1984). Arch Ophthalmol 102:520–526, © 1984, American Medical Association.)

nancy was important in predicting the severity at the end of or after pregnancy. These authors found that the rate of progression was higher in women who had background retinopathy than in women with either no retinopathy or with more advanced disease when first examined (13).

Current age or age at the time of the examination has been found to be related to the severity of retinopathy (14). In the WESDR, persons who were less than 13 years of age at the time of the examination had a rate of retinopathy that was about half that of those who were older than 13 at the time of the examination. Even after allowing for the duration of diabetes, age at examination appears to be a significant, although less important, factor (15). Other factors related to retinopathy are the presence of proteinuria and the levels of blood pressure and glycosylated hemoglobin (9).

The question often arises whether previous pregnancies are themselves a risk factor for the development or progression of diabetic retinopathy. To investigate this question, 397 women with insulin-dependent diabetes were studied. Of these women, 197 had never been pregnant, 88 had been pregnant once, 56 had been pregnant twice, and 56 had been pregnant three or more times after diabetes was diagnosed. Although the number of pregnancies was positively associated with the severity of diabetic retinopathy, when the duration of diabetes was taken into account, this relationship was no longer apparent (16) (Table 5.1). Thus, when performing a study specifically geared to current pregnancy, a history of previous pregnancy does not appear to be a risk factor.

TABLE 5.1. Distribution of women according to severity of retinopathy in the worse eye and to the number of pregnancies* (Wisconsin Health Service Area 1, September 1980 through July 1982).

Retinopathy group[†]	No. of pregnancies			
	0	1	2	3+
1	42 (21.3)[‡]	17 (19.3)	9 (16.1)	3 (5.4)
2	77 (39.1)	36 (40.9)	16 (28.6)	18 (32.1)
3	41 (20.1)	13 (14.8)	9 (16.1)	16 (28.6)
4	37 (18.8)	22 (25.0)	22 (39.3)	19 (33.9)
Total	197 (100)	88 (100)	56 (100)	56 (100)

*$\chi^2_9 p < .025$
[†]Group 1 = no retinopathy; 2 = mild nonproliferative retinopathy; 3 = hemorrhages and/or microaneurysms; 4 = proliferative retinopathy.
[‡]Percentage of women is shown in parentheses.
Reprinted with permission from Klein BEK, Klein R (1984) Gravidity and diabetic retinopathy. Am J Epidemiol 119:564–569.

Considerations for Study Design

Part of the difficulty involved in studying retinopathy during pregnancy is that youth-onset insulin-dependent diabetes is a relatively uncommon condition. In a survey of an 11-county area in south central Wisconsin between 1979 and 1981, of the 839,324 residents identified, 1,092 had insulin-dependent diabetes. Slightly more than half of these were male (17); some were women not of childbearing age. Thus, we are dealing with an uncommon disease. Many studies have been hampered by this problem. In trying to assess the influence of pregnancy on the severity of diabetic retinopathy, many studies have failed to include a comparison group, that is, a group of nonpregnant diabetic women. Variable follow-up schedules add further difficulties in trying to compare results between or even within studies. The lack of objective records of the diabetic retinopathy presents another problem, as the clinical description of retinopathy has been shown to be unreliable (18). Even when the observers are ophthalmologists, albeit with no special training in retinal disorders, the error rates in diagnosing retinopathy are high (18).

At the University of Wisconsin a study to evaluate the effects of pregnancy on retinopathy was designed with some of these shortcomings in mind. The study included two groups of insulin-dependent diabetic women: one pregnant and one not. The groups are of similar duration of diabetes, degree of retinopathy at the beginning of the observation period, and current age. These factors were chosen because they are the ones that most strongly influence the subsequent development and/or the progression of diabetic retinopathy in the absence of pregnancy. Pregnant patients are seen in the first trimester. They are then seen again in the third trimester and once again in the postpartum period. Members of the comparison group are seen at equivalent time intervals (19).

The evaluation includes obtaining a medical history, measuring blood pressure, height and weight, blood glucose and glycosylated hemoglobin, and testing urine for glucose and protein. The ophthalmologic examination consists of a refraction and visual acuity measurement done according to the Early Treatment of Diabetic Retinopathy Study protocol, slit lamp examination, intraocular pressure measurement, ophthalmoscopy, stereo fundus photography of the posterior pole, and red reflex photography. The fundus photographs are graded at the Fundus Photography Reading Center of the University of Wisconsin in Madison. A preliminary analysis, based on 140 participants (20), indicates that the groups were similar with respect to age, duration of diabetes, and severity of retinopathy. Of the 70 pregnant women, 25 had more severe retinopathy at their postpartum visit than they had had when they were first seen. Only 15 of the 70 nonpregnant women were worse after an equivalent period of time. In seven of the 70 pregnant women, the retinopathy had improved at the postpartum visit, whereas 21 of the 70 nonpregnant women showed a similar improvement. This somewhat greater tendency for the retinopathy to progress in pregnant women was apparent even after taking into account the duration of diabetes and the levels of blood pressure and glycosylated hemoglobin. Because the sample size is still quite small, it is not possible to draw firm conclusions from those data.

The Role of Glycemic Control in Pregnancy

If it is found that pregnancy appears to increase the risk of retinopathy, might that increased risk be due to a change in the degree of metabolic control occurring during the pregnancy, or might it be due to the pregnancy itself? In studies done in Denmark (21) and the United States (22), diabetic retinopathy actually appeared to worsen when the patients' blood glucose levels were acutely brought under tight control. Both of these studies were performed on small numbers of persons, and long-term follow-up is not available. Jampol et al reported that the severity of retinopathy appeared to worsen more in women whose blood glucose levels were tightly controlled during the pregnancy than in those whose blood glucose levels were less vigorously controlled (23). That study, too, was performed on a small number of persons. It remains to be seen whether this finding can be confirmed, and if so, whether vigorous control is responsible for an apparent progression of retinopathy during pregnancy. It is also uncertain whether the specific retinal changes that were found in those studies (an increase in cotton-wool patches and in intraretinal microvascular abnormalities) portend a worsening of the retinopathy after the pregnancy or whether they tend to regress. It has been found that some of these lesions themselves tend to disappear with time. These are important considerations in light of evidence that tight glucose control has beneficial effects on the fetus (24).

When to Treat Diabetic Retinopathy in Pregnancy

With regard to the individual patient, decisions need to be made even though information is imperfect. In nonpregnant women the recommendations that were outlined after the completion of the Diabetic Retinopathy Study have been followed closely (12). Therefore, in patients who have significant neovascularization of the optic nervehead, and in those with any neovascularization in the presence of vitreous hemorrhage, we recommend panretinal photocoagulation treatment. However, in pregnant patients many clinicians resort to earlier treatment (25,26). Not all physicians feel comfortable with the latter management strategy, and many prefer not to extend the indications for laser treatment beyond those suggested by the Diabetic Retinopathy Study. However, these practitioners tend to watch their patients very carefully so that treatment may be given at the earliest sign of progression, according to Diabetic Retinopathy Study Guidelines. As with all diseases and treatments in medicine, the follow-up and specific care must be geared to the individual patient. This will be true even when the importance of pregnancy in the progression of retinopathy will have been determined.

Acknowledgments. This work was supported in part by grants EY 03843 from the National Eye Institute, National Institutes of Health, and from a grant from the Retina Research Foundation.

The author wishes to thank Dr. Ronald Klein for advice during various stages of the research project and Mae Wildt for manuscript preparation.

References

1. Coustan DR (1985) Management of the Pregnant Diabetic. In: Olefsky JM, Sherwin RS (eds) Diabetes Mellitus: Management and Complications. Churchill Livingstone, New York, Edinburgh, London, and Melbourne, pp 311.
2. White P (1965) Pregnancy and diabetes, Medical Aspects. Med Clin North Am 49:1015–1024.
3. Cassar J, Kohner EM, Hamilton AM, Gordon H, Joplin GF (1978) Diabetic retinopathy and pregnancy. Diabetologia 15:105–111.
4. Jervell J, Moe J, Skjaeraasen, Blystad W, Egge K (1979) Diabetes mellitus and pregnancy—management and results at Rikshospitalet, Oslo, 1970–1977. Diabetologia 16:151–155.
5. Frank RN, Hoffman WH, Podgor MJ (1982) Retinopathy in juvenile-onset type I diabetes of short duration. Diabetes 31:874–882.
6. Palmberg P, Smith M, Waltman S (1981) The Material history of retinopathy in insulin-dependent juvenile-onset diabetes. Ophthalmology 88:613–618.
7. White P (1960) Childhood diabetes. Diabetes 9:345.
8. Kornerup T (1955) Studies in diabetic retinopathy: An investigation of 1000 cases of diabetes. Acta Med Scand 153:81–101.
9. Klein R, Klein BEK, Moss SE, Davis MD, DeMets DL (1984) The Wisconsin Epidemiologic Study of Diabetic Retinopathy II. Prevalence and risk of diabetic retinopathy when age at diagnosis is less than 30 years. Arch Ophthalmol 102:520–526.
10. Klein R, Klein BEK, Moss SE, Davis MD, DeMets DL (1984) The Wisconsin Epidemiologic Study of Diabetic Retinopathy III. Prevalence and risk of diabetic retinopathy when age at diagnosis is 30 or more years. Arch Ophthalmol 102: 527–532.
11. Klein BEK, Davis MD, Segal P, Long JA, Harris WA, Haug GA, Magli YL, Syrjala S (1984) Diabetic retinopathy. Assessment of severity and progression. Ophthalmology 91:10–17.
12. The Diabetic Retinopathy Study Research Group (1978) Photocoagulation treatment of proliferative diabetic retinopathy: the second report of Diabetic Retinopathy Study findings. Ophthalmology 85:82–106.

13. Horvat M, Maclean H, Goldberg L, Crock GW (1980) Diabetic retinopathy in pregnancy: a 12 year prospective survey. Br J Opthalmol 64:398–403.
14. Burditt AF, Caird FL, Draper GJ (1968) The natural history of diabetic retinopathy. Quart J Med 37:303–317.
15. Klein R, Klein BEK, Moss SE, Davis MD, DeMets DL (1985) Retinopathy in Young-onset diabetic patients. Diabetes Care 8:311–315.
16. Klein BEK, Klein R (1984) Gravidity and diabetic retinopathy. AM J Epidemiol 119:564–569.
17. Klein R, Klein BEK, Moss SE, DeMets DL, Kaufman I, Voss C (1984) Prevalence of diabetes mellitus in southern Wisconsin. Am J Epidemiol 119:54–61.
18. Sussman EJ, Tsiaras WG, Soper KA (1982) Diagnosis of diabetic eye disease. JAMA 247:3231–3234.
19. Klein BEK, Klein R (1983) The retinopathy in pregnancy study: Rationale and design. Invest Ophthalmol Vis Sci [Suppl] 26:85.
20. Klein BEK, Klein R (1985) Retinopathy in the pregnant diabetic patient: A preliminary report. Abstracts of the Second NEI Symposium on Eye Disease Epidemiology, USDHHS, National Eye Institute, National Institutes of Health, Bethesda, Maryland.
21. Lauritzen T, Frost-Larsen K, Larsen HW, Deckert T (1983) Effect of 1 yer of near-normal blood glucose levels on retinopathy in insulin-dependent diabetics. Lancet 1:200–204.
22. Kroc Collaborative Study Group (1984) Blood glucose control and the evolution of diabetic retinopathy and albuminuria. N Engl J Med 311:365–372.
23. Jampol LM, Phelps R, Sakol P, Metzger B, Feinkel N (1986) Diabetic retinopathy during pregnancy: role of regulation of hyperglycemia. Invest Ophthalmol Vis Sci [Suppl] 27:4.
24. Ylinen K, Raivio K, Teramo K (1981) Hemoglobin AlC predicts the perinatal outcome in insulin-dependent diabetic pregnancies. Br J Obstet Gynecol 88:961–967.
25. Cassar J, Kohner EM, Hamilton AM, Gordon H, Joplin GF (1978) Diabetic retinopathy and pregnancy. Diabetologia 15:105–111.
26. Hercules BL, Wozencroft M, Gayed IL, Jeacock J (1980) Peripheral retinal ablation in the treatment of proliferative diabetic retinopathy during pregnancy. Br J Opthalmol 64:87–93.

6
Thyroid Disorders in Pregnant Women With Type I Diabetes

Lois Jovanovic and Charles M. Peterson

Introduction

The association of diabetes with thyroid disorders is well documented (1–9). The incidence of clinical and subclinical thyroid disorders in patients with type I diabetes (insulin-dependent diabetes or IDD) has been reported to be as high as 30% (10). The incidence of hypothyroidism in a diabetic population varies from 0.2% to 12%, with a female prevalence over males as high as 7:1 (2). Hyperthyrodism may also be increased in patients with insulin-dependent diabetes mellitus, with a ratio of females to males between 2 and 5:1 (9). If the prevalence of thyroid dysfunction is so high in women with diabetes mellitus, then the clinician who cares for pregnant women (up to 20% with thyroid problems), type I diabetic (up to 30% with thyroid problems) women (sevenfold increase in prevalence over males) should be especially aware of the strategies for diagnosis and management of thyroid disorders. This chapter briefly reviews the literature concerning thyroid disease and type I diabetes, thyroid disease and pregnancy, and the occurrence of all three together. It also suggests surveillance and treatment protocols for managing the thyroid problems that complicate pregnancies in the woman with IDD.

Diabetes Mellitus and Thyroid Disorders

As suggested above, if the clinical and subclinical thyroid disorders found in IDD patients are taken together, the incidence may approach 30% (10). Sugrue et al (11) retrospectively evaluated 5,000 diabetic patients of whom 950 had hyperthyroidism (19%) and 500 had hypothyroidism (10%) for a combined prevalence of 29%. Their female to male ratio was 4.6:1 for hyperthyroidism and 7.1:1 for hypothyroidism.

The prevalence of thyroid antibodies is increased in 20% to 40% of patients with diabetes mellitus (3–7). Goldstein et al (6) detected antithyroid microsomal antibodies in 8% of pediatric diabetic patients without any clinical evidence of thyroid disease as opposed to 0.5% of the control population. Riley et al (12) screened patients with IDD and found anti-thyroid microsomal antibodies in 17% of them. Again, more females had positive titers than males. Bright et al (10) reported antibodies to thyroid in 30% of their diabetic patients.

Gray et al (2) detected elevated thyroid-stimulating hormone (TSH) values as evidence of hypothyroidism in 12% of IDD patients as compared with 6% of patients with non-insulin-dependent (NIDD) or type II diabetes and 5% of nondiabetic patients. They, too, reported that more females (17%) had evidence of hypothyroidism than males (6.1%). The observation by Sugrue et al (11) that in diabetic patients there may be progression to clinical hypothyroidism warranting treatment at a rate of 3% per year may be especially significant for the IDD woman who becomes pregnant.

Thyroid Disorders During Pregnancy

Although the occurrence of thyroid enlargement during pregnancy has been known since antiquity and immortalized in the paintings of Rubens (13), the etiology of this enlargement is still in question. Theories explaining this physiologic response include (a) relative iodine deficiency (b) TSH-like action of human chorionic gonadotropin, and (c) increased hormonal production secondary to the increased metabolic demand of pregnancy (14).

Even when pregnant women are clinically euthyroid, numerous changes can be detected using tests of thyroid function. There is a 20% increase in the basal metabolic rate in normal pregnancy (15). Free thyroid hormone levels are reported to be normal, but because pregnancy-related elevations in serum estrogen levels increase the liver production of thyroid-binding globulins, and because thyroid hormones are more than 99% protein bound, protein-bound iodine (PBI), total serum thyroxine (T_4), triiodothyronine (T_3), and reverse $(3,3',5')$ triiodothyronine (rT_3) may appear elevated.

Total thyroid hormone concentration increases to maximal levels in the second trimester and usually returns to normal during the first month after delivery (16). Steady-state thyroxine turnover and urinary free T_3 and T_4 are unaltered during pregnancy (17). Thyroid-stimulating hormone levels are slightly elevated during the first trimester (21), but revert to normal thereafter (18).

The reported frequency of hyperthyroidism occurring de novo during pregnancy has varied from 0.5% to 3% (19,20). Sugrue and Drury (21) reported a frequency of 0.05% in a population of 72,250. The diagnosis of hyperthyroidism may be difficult during pregnancy because the usual presenting symptoms of hyperthyroidism such as anxiety, insomnia, palpitations, dyspnea, sweating, irritability, and enlarged thyroid may occur normally in pregnancy. In addition, the pregnancy-related elevations of T_4, T_3, and rT_3 make laboratory confirmation of clinical suspicion difficult. Thus, the two most useful laboratory tests for hyperthyroidism during pregnancy are measurement of the free T_4 and the monoclonal antibody "extra-sensitive" assay of TSH.

An accurate diagnosis is important because untreated hyperthyroidism is associated with increased fetal loss, premature labor, and intrauterine growth retardation (22). There is some evidence that thyrotoxicosis may be ameliorated during pregnancy (23,24) perhaps as a result of the decrease in fluid and cellular immunity; but because the risk to the fetus is so great, definitive treatment is advocated. We therefore offer a protocol for the screening of all pregnant women for thyroid dysfunction. We suggest that T_4 and TSH be measured at the time of the first visit of the pregnancy, and if the TSH is too high or too low, diagnostic tests should be ordered (Table 6.1).

On the other hand, a decrease in fertility occurs with hypothyroidism. In a review of the literature, Montoro et al (25) found only 36 cases of pregnancy in clinically hypothyroid women. Weight gain, fatigue, constipation, hair and skin changes are classic signs not only of pregnancy, but of hypothyroidism as well. Thus, laboratory confirmation of a clinical impression is always necessary (Table 6.1). Pregnancy raises the plasma concentration of T_4. Thus, a "normal" or "low normal T_4" may, in fact, be abnormal for a pregnant woman and the extra-sensitive measurement of TSH and/or a free T_4 hormone determination is needed to interpret the significance of the total T_4 values (Table 6.1).

TABLE 6.1. Flow diagram for the screening and diagnosis of thyroid dysfunction during pregnancy.

Screening tests:	Total T_4 and TSH[a]		
	"Normal T_4" elevated TSH	"Elevated" T_4 and nl TSH	Elevated T_4 and low TSH
Diagnostic tests:	*Hypothyroidism* Free T_4 RIA Free T_3 RIA	*Normal thyroid function* Free T_4 RIA Repeat TSH at 20 weeks or if 24-h urine for protein is elevated	*Hyperthyroidism* Confirm with Free T_4 RIA Free T_3 RIA

[a]Measured with monoclonal antibody.

Thyroid Disorders in Diabetic Pregnant Women

The preceding discussion leads to the conclusion that being female, pregnant, and diabetic increase the risk of thyroid dysfunction. Indeed, Soler and Nicholson (26) reported a 20% incidence of clinically significant thyroid disease in a group of pregnant patients with juvenile onset diabetes. In fact, with the advent of programs that achieve normoglycemia during pregnancy (27), thyroid disease may become the most common complication of diabetes in pregnancy.

We studied the incidence not only of clinically significant thyroid disease, but also of subclinical thyroid disease as manifested by a normal T_4 but abnormal antithyroid antibody titers and/or an elevated TSH in 51 pregnant women with IDD (C-peptide $<$ 0.03 pg/mL). At 6, 12, 18, and 24 weeks of gestation, we measured T_4, TSH, antimicrosomal and antithyroid antibodies, 24-hour urine for creatinine clearance, and total urinary protein. Eight of the 51 patients (16%) developed hypothyroidism during the study. All eight had a normal T_4 at 6 weeks, but had positive antibody titers and/or a TSH above 4.0 μU/mL (normal $<$ 4.0). They also had proteinuria ($>$ 4.0 g/24 h). The eight women all developed hypothyroidism between 18 and 24 weeks of gestation. During the first trimester, the overall rate of subclinical thyroid disease, defined by at least one abnormal laboratory test, was slightly above 50% in these 51 women who were clinically euthyroid and had a normal T_4 at the beginning of gestation.

The insulin requirement of the eight patients with new onset hypothyroidism fell at about 20 $\pm$ 2 weeks of the pregnancy. Thus, hypothyroidism appears to be an additional cause of decreased insulin requirement during gestation—a requirement that otherwise tends to remain relatively uniform at this period in pregnancies complicated by diabetes. Other causes of dropping insulin requirement are decreased food consumption and consequent weight loss, increased exercise, failing placenta, and/or decreasing renal function. Since these eight women maintained adequate renal function despite massive proteinuria, and since food intake and weight remained appropriate for gestational age, and fetal well-being was documented, hypothyroidism appeared to be the probable cause of the decreased insulin requirement.

When we looked at such variables as duration of diabetes, proteinuria, TSH, insulin requirement, and T_4 at 24 weeks, the only correlation that emerged in this population of 51 pregnant women with IDD was between duration of diabetes and degree of proteinuria during pregnancy (Figure 6.1).

A significant correlation ($r = +.81$, $p<.001$) between the degree of proteinuria and the daily excretion of thyroxine-binding globulin, and between the degree of proteinuria and daily T_4 loss ($r = +.53$, $p<.001$) has been reported in ten men with nephrotic syndrome and a mean urinary excretion of T_4 of 69 mg/d (28). Thus, the increased prevalence of hypothyroidism seen in our study may have been due partly to the inability of an already

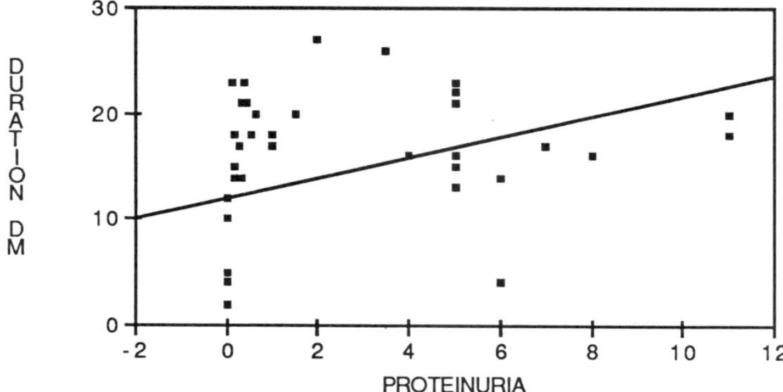

FIGURE 6.1. Correlation between duration of diabetes (DM) in years and degree of protein excretion over 24 hours (g/24 h). $r = .4, p < .01$.

immunologically damaged thyroid to handle increased hormonal production necessitated by the pregnancy and partly to the urinary loss of T_4. Mogensen (29) noted that when massive proteinuria occurs, large molecular weight proteins are lost. Malins (30) agreed that once massive proteinuria occurs in diabetic nephropathy, there is no characteristic pattern of protein excretion. Thus a 40-fold increase in proteinuria secondary to diabetic nephropathy exacerbated by pregnancy, as seen in our eight patients, could have caused a marked urinary loss of T_4 since 12% of T_4 and 9% of T_3 in normal urine are bound to proteins (31).

Hyperthyroidism occurring de novo in pregnant women with IDD appears to be quite rare. Sugrue and Drury mention having seen three cases (21). We have not seen a case complicated by type I diabetes in more than 300 pregnancies. The reason for this phenomenon in a population otherwise at risk is poorly understood, but may reflect the ameliorating effects of pregnancy on the antibody and cellular components of the immune system.

Treatment of Thyroid Disease During Pregnancy in Women With IDD

It is apparent from the above discussion that hypothyroid disease is the more common complicating thyroid illness during pregnancy in women with IDD. Treatment should begin with thyroid replacement as soon as the laboratory values verify the clinical impression (Table 6.1). L-Thyroxine is recommended as the treatment of choice for it allows direct monitoring by means of serum T_4 levels, gives a constant serum concentration of T_4, allows peripheral conversion of T_4 to T_3 as needed, and has a half-life of 18 to 24 hours compared with a T_3 half-life of 6 to 8 hours.

The recommended replacement dose of L-thyroxine varies between 0.1 and 0.2 mg/d. We suggest that the starting dose be 0.2 mg/d. The usual clinical parameters of thyroid function (tachycardia, nervousness, palpitations, sweating, reflexes) cannot be used to titrate the dose of L-thyroxine because these clinical signs occur frequently in normal pregnancy. Thyroid-stimulating hormone may take up to 2 weeks to normalize, once euthyroidism has been achieved. Therefore, L-thyroxine could be overprescribed if the clinician were to increase the dose until the TSH fell. On the other hand, following our observation that the insulin requirement is inappropriately low, we adjust the dose of L-thyroxine until we reach the desired insulin requirement (0.7 U/kg/24 h from weeks 6 to 12; 0.8 U/kg/24 h from weeks 13 to 24; 0.9 U/kg/24 h for weeks 25 to 36; and 1.0 U/kg/24 h, for weeks 37 to term) (27). Thyroid tests (T_4 and TSH) should be repeated at 2- to 3-week intervals after starting the dose and should be normal 2 to 3 weeks after the insulin requirement becomes appropriate for gestational age.

The neonatal outcome of hypothyroid patients is good (32), probably because the fetal hypothalamic-pituitary-thyroid axis develops and functions independently of the maternal axis, and these hormones do not generally cross the placenta (18). Congenital thyroid disease is not a neonatal complication of infants born to mothers with hypothyroidism, except in areas of endemic goiter, where iodine insufficiency affects mother and fetus, independently.

Hyperthyroid disease in a pregnant diabetic woman must also be treated. Radioactive iodine is contraindicated because it crosses the placenta and is concentrated in the fetal thyroid. Iodides and potassium perchlorate are contraindicated for the same reasons. Surgery, although not interfering with fetal hormone production, is not favored because of the risks of maternal hypoparathyroidism, anesthesia, and blood loss (33). Three groups of drugs have been found effective: thiouracils, imidazoles, and β-adrenergic blockers. However, all of these drugs cross the placenta (34,35) and thus can interfere with fetal thyroid function. Because of the limited permeability of the placenta to T_4, giving an antithyroid drug with L-thyroxine to the mother is not guaranteed to prevent hypothyroidism in the infant (36).

Thiouracils prevent iodine binding to thyroid hormone precursors and decrease the peripheral conversion of T_4 to T_3. The thiouracil most commonly used in the United States is propylthiouracil (PTU). The usual daily dose is 200 to 300 mg in three equal dosages given eight hours apart then decreased to 50 to 150 mg a day. Excretion of the drug in maternal milk occurs, and the side effects of gastrointestinal upset, skin rash, and depression of bone marrow must be monitored closely. Although the thiouracils do not affect either insulin pharmacokinetics or glucose tolerance, the normalization of thyroid function reduces the insulin requirement to a level more appropriate to the gestational age.

Carbimazole is the imidazole derivative most commonly used outside the United States. This drug is concentrated in both maternal and fetal thyroid glands (37). It may also inhibit the production of thyroid antibodies (38). The initial dose is 40 to 60 mg every six hours, which is then decreased to 5 to 15 mg a day. Imidazoles are also excreted into maternal milk. These drugs, like the thiouracils, do not affect glucose levels directly but, since they improve thyroid function, they reduce the insulin requirement to normal.

Propranolol antagonizes the sympathomimetic effects of thyroid hormones and stimulates the conversion of T_4 to rT_3. There are only eight reported cases in which propranolol was used as the sole treatment of hyperthyroidism during pregnancy and they all ended with normal births. (39,40) However, the use of propranolol for other medical problems during gestation (arrhythmias, mitral valve prolapse, hypertension), may cause fetal bradycardia, intrauterine growth retardation, neonatal hypoglycemia, and respiratory distress syndrome (41,42). Propranolol also is excreted into the milk. Propranolol decreases insulin secretion and may therefore cause deterioration of the glucose tolerance in a diabetic woman under dietary management, or it may increase the insulin requirement in a woman with residual insulin secretion. Propranolol also blunts the warning signs of hypoglycemia and therefore may be dangerous for an IDD woman.

As can be seen, there is a lack of unanimity concerning the treatment of choice for hyperthyroidism during pregnancy, much less pregnancy complicated by diabetes. All thyroidologists agree that the ideal drug would be one that adequately treats maternal hyperthyroidism with minimal maternal side effects and without interfering with the fetal pituitary-thyroid axis. Unfortunately, to date, there is no such drug. We have therefore chosen to review three treatment programs that have resulted in the best maternal-fetal outcome.

Sugrue and Drury in Dublin (21) have a series of 73 patients with hyperthyroidism complicating pregnancy and a fetal loss rate of 13.4%, compared with losses of 14% to 33% reported by others using other drug regimens. They recommend a maintenance dose of carbimazole 5 to 10 mg a day for patients diagnosed for the first time during pregnancy. They recommend an initial dosage of 15 mg four times a day, to be tapered over 6 to 8 weeks to a daily maintenance dose of 5 to 10 mg. Treatment should be stopped at 37 weeks and resumed immediately after delivery, with breast-feeding prohibited.

Mestman (43) favors PTU starting at 300 to 400 mg a day in three divided doses. Once improvement occurs, the amount of the drug should be halved. If improvement persists, the drug should continue to be tapered to 100 mg a day. Mestman recommends that if the patient remains euthyroid for approximately 4 to 6 weeks on the minimum amount of drug, PTU be discontinued as long as the thyroid function tests done every 2 weeks remain normal.

Momotani et al (38) compared fetal and maternal serum indices of thyroid function in 70 patients with hyperthyroidism and noted a strong correlation between fetal and maternal T_4 levels in the women who continued PTU throughout pregnancy and in those who discontinued such treatment. This observation suggests that the fetal thyroid is under the same stimulatory or inhibitory influence as the maternal thyroid and, therefore, that the function of the maternal thyroid is a useful index of fetal thyroid status. A significant correlation was found also between maternal levels of antithyrotropin-binding antibodies and fetal levels of T_4 after PTU treatment was stopped, suggesting that the maternal antibody titer is a useful index of the fetal need for continued treatment of the mother with PTU.

They concluded that serial measurements of maternal T_4, and antithyrotropin-binding antibodies are useful guides for monitoring therapy. The PTU dosage that maintains maternal T_4 in a mildly thyrotoxic range was considered appropriate for maintaining euthyroidism in the fetus, for although the neonates had no signs or symptoms of hypothyroidism, there was a significant inverse correlation between thyrotropin and T_4 levels in the fetuses of mothers who continued taking thionamides, suggesting that a low fetal T_4 level is evidence of fetal hypothyroidism. The higher incidence of combined low T_4 and high thyrotropin levels in the fetuses than in the mothers indicates that a dose of thionamides sufficient to maintain maternal T_4 levels within the normal range is somewhat excessive for the fetus. These findings corroborate the widely held belief that in order to prevent fetal hypothyroidism, pregnant women with thyrotoxicosis should be treated with the lowest doses of an antithyroid drug that can maintain the maternal levels of thyroid hormone in the upper normal or slightly thyrotoxic range.

Thyroid storm is a rare complication of labor and/or cesarean section and, as noted above, is probably even more rare when pregnancy is complicated by diabetes (44). Treatment of thyroid storm should include treatment of infection, rehydration, correction of hyperthermia, anticonvulsant therapy, iodine administration, increased PTU dosage, and the use of propranolol and corticosteroids just as would be done in a pregnant individual without diabetes mellitus. All the while glucose levels must be held within the normal range by hourly bedside blood glucose monitoring and adjustment of the intravenous infusion of insulin.

The thyroid function of infants born to well-managed hypothyroid mothers is excellent (35). However, a long-term follow-up of infants born with signs of hypothyroidism showed that 35% of them remained hypothyroid, 27% had psychomotor abnormalities, and 42% had some retardation of skeletal growth. Momotani et al (45) looked at the relationship between first trimester maternal hyperthyroidism and subsequent congenital malformations in the offspring. In those mothers who were hyperthyroid at the time of conception, the malformation rate was 3% compared with 0.2% in a group of euthyroid mothers. These findings show that it is probably uncontrolled hyperthyroidism per se that results in malformations of the offspring and that its rate can be decreased with the use of antithyroid drugs. The interaction of hyperthyroidism and diabetes on the prevalence of malformations has not been studied.

Conclusion

In summary, IDD is associated with a 20% risk of thyroid dysfunction. Pregnancy may further increase this risk. Risk factors that can predict which women will develop clinically significant thyroid dysfunction during pregnancy include proteinuria > 4 g/24 h and evidence of an elevated TSH and/or antimicrosomal or antithyroid antibodies despite a normal T_4 at the start of pregnancy. It is suggested, therefore, that a 24-hour urine examination for proteinuria and appropriate thyroid function tests (T_4, TSH, and antibodies) be a part of the assessment of women with IDD during gestation as well as before.

References

1. Irvine WJ (1979) Autoimmunity in endocrine disease. Clin Endocrinol Metab 4:227–235.
2. Gray RS, Dorsey DQ, Seth J, et al (1980) Prevalence of subclinical thyroid failure in insulin dependent diabetes. J Clin Endocrinol Metab 50:1034–1045.
3. Landing BH, Pettit MD, Wiens RL, et al (1964) Schmidt's syndrome (thyroid and adrenal insufficiency). A review of the literature and report of 15 new cases including 10 instances of coexistent diabetes mellitus. Medicine 43:153–162.
4. Ungar B, Stocks AE, Martin FIR, et al (1968) Intrinsic-factor antibody, parietal-cell antibody, and latent pernicious anemia in diabetes mellitus. Lancet 1:415–416.
5. Irvine WJ, Scarth L, Clarke BF, et al (1970) Thyroid and gastric autoimmunity in patients with diabetes mellitus. Lancet 1:163–165.
6. Goldstein DE, Drash A, Gibbs J, Blizzard RM (1970) Diabetes mellitus: The incidence of circulation antibodies against thyroid, gastric and adrenal tissue. J Pediatr 77:304–309.
7. Nerup J, Binder C (1973) Thyroid, gastric and adrenal autoimmunity in diabetes mellitus. Acta Endocrinol 72:279–285.
8. Fialkow PJ, Zavala C, Nielsen R (1975) Thyroid autoimmunity: Increase frequency in relatives of insulin-dependent diabetic patients. Ann Intern Med 83:170–174.
9. Cooppan R, Kozak GP (1980) Hyperthyroidism and diabaetes mellitus. An analysis of 70 patients. Arch Intern Med 140:370–377.
10. Bright GM, Blizzard RM, Kaiser DI, et al (1982) Organ-specific autoantibodies in children with common endocrine diseases. J Pediatr 100:8–12.
11. Sugrue DD, McEvoy M, Drury MI (1982) Thyroid disease in diabetics. Postgrad Med J 58:680–684.

12. Riley WJ, MacClaren NK, Lezzote DC, et al (1981) Thyroid autoimmunity in insulin diabetes mellitus: The case for routine screening. J Pediatr 98:350–356.
13. Jovanovic L, Subak-Sharpe G (1987) The woman's answer book. Athenium, New York.
14. Jovanovic L, Singh M, Saxena BB, et al (1987) Verification of early pregnancy tests in a multicenter trial. Proc Soc Exp Biol Med 184:201–205, 1987.
15. Mussey RD (1938) Changes in basal metabolic rate during pregnancy. Am J Obstet Gynecol 36:59–65.
16. Amino N, Mari H, Iwatani Y, et al (1982) High prevalence of transient postpartum thyroitoricosis and hypothyroidism, N Engl J Med 306:849–853.
17. Burrow GN (1975) Pregnancy and thyroid function, Med Clin North Am. 59:1089–1109.
18. Tulchinsky D, Ryan KJ (1980) Maternal Fetal Endocrinology, WB Saunders, Toronto, pp 115–128.
19. Silver S. (1960) The thyroid gland, medical surgical and gynecological complications of pregnancy, ed 2, in Guttmacher AF, Rovinsky JJ (eds). Williams & Wilkins, Baltimore, pp 561–582.
20. Mussey RD, Haines SF, Ward E (1948) Pregnancy and hyperthyroidism. Am J Obstet Gynecol 55:609–615.
21. Sugrue D, Drury MI (1980) Hyperthyroidism complicating pregnancy: results of treatment by antithyroid drugs in 77 pregnancies. Br J Obstet Gynecol 87:970–975.
22. Drury MI (1986) Hyperthyroidism in pregnancy. J R Soc Med 79:317–319.
23. Jonckheer MH, Decostre P, Bastenie PA (1976) Amelioration of hyperthyroidism during pregnancy. Rev Gynecol Obstet 71:205–210.
24. Serup J, Peterson S (1977) Improvement of Grave's disease during pregnancy. Acta Obstet Gynecol Scand 56:463–468.
25. Montoro M, Collea JV, Frasier SD, et al (1981) Successful outcome of pregnancy in women with hypothyroidism. Ann Intern Med 94:31–39.
26. Soler NG, Nicholson H (1979) Diabetes and thyroid disease during pregnancy. Obstet Gynecol 54:18–23.
27. Jovanovic L, Druzin M, Peterson CMP (1981) The effect of euglycemia on the outcome of pregnancy in insulin-dependent diabetics as compared to normal controls. Am J Med 71:921–927.
28. Gavin LA, McMahon FA, Castle JN, et al (1978) Alterations in serum thyroid and thyroxine-binding globulin in patients with nephrosis. J Clin Endocrin Metab 1:125–32.
29. Mogensen CE (1981) Abnormal physiological processes in the kidney in Handbook of Diabetes Mellitus. Biochemical Pathology. Brownlee M (ed). STPM Press, New York, pp 23–25.
30. Malins J (1968) Clinical Diabetes Mellitus. Ergro & Spottiswoode, London.
31. Burke CW, Shakespear RA (1976) Triiodthyronine and thyroxine in urine. II. Renal handling and effect of urinary protein. J Clin Endocrinol Metab 42:504–510.
32. Mann EB (1975) Maternal hypothyroxinemia, development of 4 and 7 years old offspring, in Fisher DA, Burrows GN (eds): Perinatal thyroid physiology and disease. Raven Press, New York, pp 117–136.
33. Edis AJ (1979) Prevention and management of complications associated with thyroid and parathyroid surgery. Surg Clin North Am 59:83–86.

34. Selenkow HA (1972) Antithyroid-thyroid therapy of thyrotoxicosis during pregnancy. Obstet Gynecol 40:117–123.
35. Mestman JH (1981) Diagnosis and management of hyperthyroidism in pregnancy. Curr Probl Obstet Gynecol 4:10–20.
36. Ramsay I, Kaur S, Krassas G (1983) Thyrotoxicosis in pregnancy: Results of treatment by antithyroid drugs combined with T_4. Clin Endocrinol 18:73–82.
37. Drury MI, Sugrue DD, Drury RM (1984) A review of thyroid disease in pregnancy. Clin Exp Obstet Gynecol 3:79–84.
38. Momotani N, Jaeduk N, Hiroshi O, et al (1986) Antithyroid drug therapy for graves' disease during pregnancy: Optimal regimen for fetal thyroid status. N Engl J Med 315:24–28.
39. Turnstall ME (1969) The effect of propranolol on the onset of breathing at birth. Br J Anaesth 41:792–795.
40. Bullock JL, Harris RE, Young R (1975) Propranolol as the sole treatment for Graves' disease during pregnancy. 121:242–248.
41. Gladstone GR, Hordof A, Gersony WM (1975) Use of propranolol during pregnancy. J Pediatr 86:962–966.
42. Habib A, McCarthy JS (1977) Neonatal morbidity with the use of propranolol during pregnancy. J Pediatr 91:808–812.
43. Mestman JH (1986) Polyglandular Autoimmune Syndrome and Throid Disorders in Pregnancy, in Jovanovic L, Peterson CM, Fuhrmann, K (eds): Diabetes and Pregnancy: Teratology, Toxicology and Treatment, Praeger, New York, pp 321–360.
44. Guenter KE, Fridland GA (1956) Thyroid storm compicating pregnancy, Obstet Gynecol 26:403–410.
45. Momotani N, Ito K. Hamada N, et al (1984) Maternal hyperthyroidism and congenital malformation in the offspring. Clin Endocrinol 20:295–299.

7
Exercise in Gestational Diabetes

Raul Artal

Introduction

Obesity and physical inactivity have been related to glucose intolerance, and, conversely, exercise has been recommended as an adjunct therapy to improve control of glycemia in diabetic patients (1,2). Pregnant diabetic women were denied this option in the past primarily because of the fear that maternal benefits could be offset by potential fetal risks. Recent studies (3) and interest have culminated in a recommendation by the Second International Workshop-Conference on Gestational Diabetes Mellitus that women with an active life-style continue a program of moderate exercise to be conducted under medical supervision (4). The aim of this chapter is to review the normal exercise physiology of pregnancy and its relevance to the pregnant diabetic woman.

Maternal Physiologic Responses to Exercise in Pregnancy

The times when pregnant women were confined and denied the freedom of physical activity are long gone. Reasonable information and proper guidelines for exercise in pregnancy are now available (5). However, exercise prescription requires a special awareness of the physical limitations imposed by pregnancy.

Anatomic Changes in Pregnancy

Some of the most profound changes occur in the ground substance and connective tissue that become less abundant and more stretchable in pregnancy. These changes occur under the influence of hormones such as relaxin. The result is ligament laxity and joint instability, rendering joints more susceptible to injury (6).

Significant changes also occur in the vertebral column in response to a continuous shift in the center of gravity. The result is progressive lordosis and kyphosis and added risk of soft-tissue injury.

Cardiovascular Adaptations to Exercise in Pregnancy

Pregnancy is characterized by major hemodynamic changes, the most significant of which are an increase in maternal blood volume (up to 30% or more), increased cardiac output, and increased heart rate. The heart rate response to exercise in pregnancy is variable, thus the use of specific target heart rates in pregnancy appears inappropriate. Because of some of the above changes, pregnant women do have a lower cardiac reserve and are limited in performing physical activities in comparison to nonpregnant women.

One major hemodynamic concern in pregnancy is that during exercise, redistribution of blood flow away from the visceral organs to the working muscles may affect oxygen transfer to the fetus. This concern is of particular relevance to the pregnant diabetic woman because of the potential existence of arteriosclerotic vascular disease that could further impair this exchange.

Exercise induces hemodynamic compensatory changes in both the pregnant and the nonpregnant woman. Among these changes are a catecholamine-mediated increase in heart rate that is inversely correlated with R-pulse intervals (Figure 7.1), reflecting the preejection period of the heart.

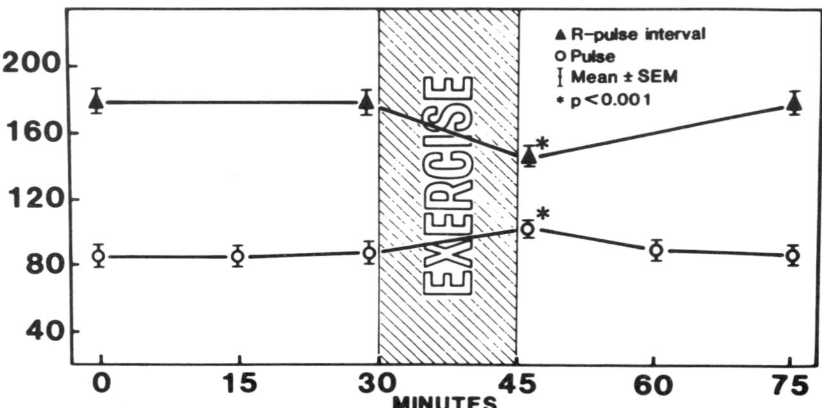

FIGURE 7.1. Comparison of the effect of exercise on the R-pulse interval (milliseconds ± 1 SEM) and on the maternal heart rate (beats per minute ± 1 SEM). The asterisk indicates a significant statistical difference for that value when compared with the preexercise value. (Reprinted with permission from Artal et al, reference 7.)

Thus, significant increases in heart rate and cardiac output, as observed during exercise, result in an increased cardiac preload and shortened R-pulse intervals. In cardiovascular disease and in diabetic patients, such compensatory responses can be significantly altered.

Pulmonary Responses to Exercise in Pregnancy

Pregnancy is characterized by significant compensatory pulmonary changes that, at rest, result in a very efficient respiratory system characterized by a state of hyperventilation primarily due to a significant increase in tidal volume (Figure 7.2). With exercise, however, this advantageous state is lost, because although ventilation increases adequately when the exercise is mild, it does not increase proportionately to moderate or severe exercise.

During rest and exercise, oxygen consumption is increased in pregnancy. However, during intense exercise, the increment is significantly lower in pregnant than in nonpregnant women (Figure 7.3).

This blunted response indicates a decrease in pulmonary reserve and an inability to compensate effectively for anaerobic exercise, as reflected in the CO_2 levels (Figure 7.4) and the respiratory exchange ratio RQ (Figure 7.5). The RQ gives an approximate estimate of which foodstuff is consumed at any given moment. During exercise in pregnancy, the RQ determinations indicate a preferential utilization of carbohydrates. This fact

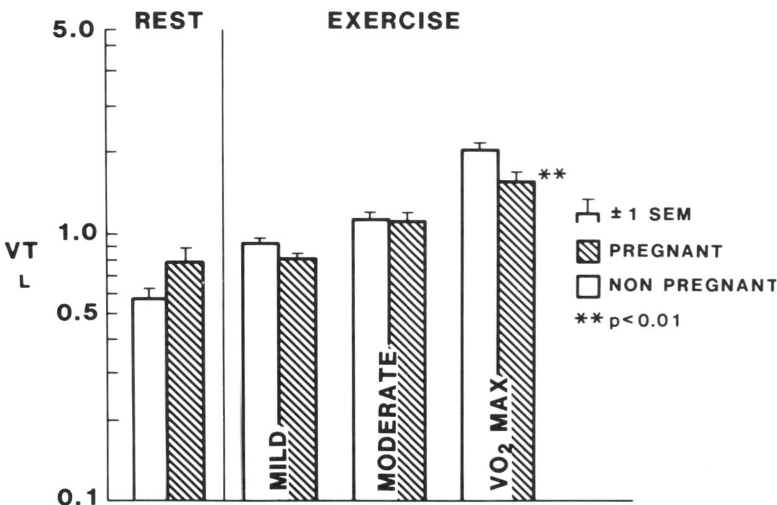

FIGURE 7.2. Tidal volume *(VT)* in liters *(L)* during rest and at the peak of mild, moderate, and maximal oxygen consumption exercise. (Reprinted with permission from Artal et al, reference 8.)

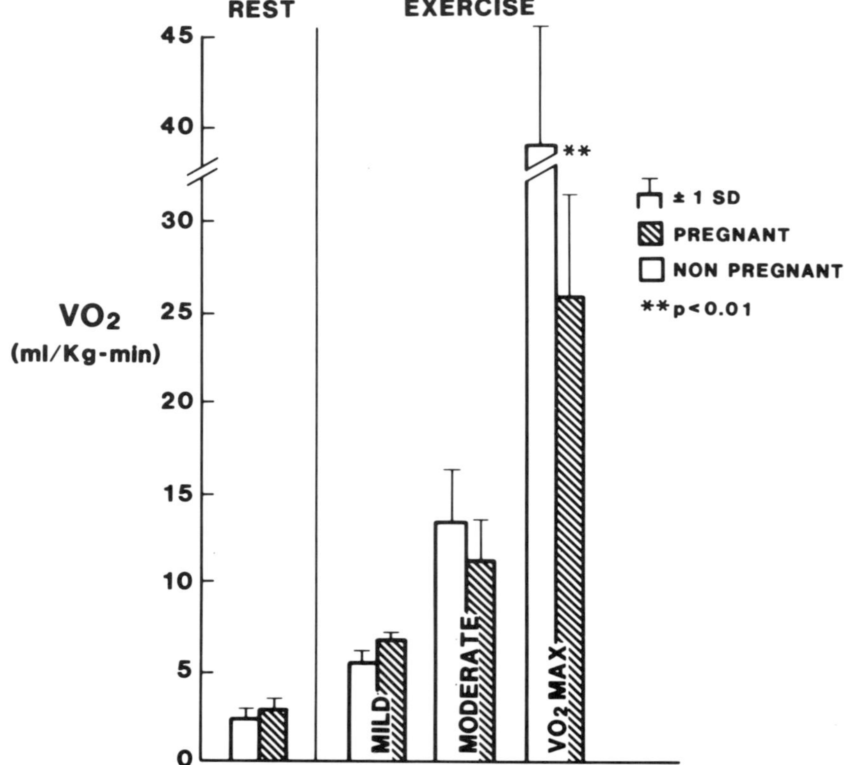

FIGURE 7.3. Oxygen consumption *(VO₂)* determinations obtained at rest and then at the peak of mild, moderate, and maximal oxygen consumption exercise. (Reprinted with permission from Artal et al, reference 8.)

is important for exercise prescription in pregnancy, for it recognizes that carbohydrate utilization could be rapid and result in undesirable episodes of hypoglycemia. Hence, pregnant women should avoid prolonged or strenuous exercise. Furthermore, individuals on insulin therapy are particularly vulnerable and should be closely supervised while exercising.

Nutritional Requirements in Pregnancy

The metabolic adaptations to pregnancy require an additional intake of 300 kcal a day. Physically active women need proportionally more. Indeed, the use of exercise to induce weight reduction should be discouraged during pregnancy because of its potentially adverse effect on the fetus, as detailed below. However, exercise can be utilized in the pregnant diabetic woman to decrease insulin resistance and maintain normoglycemia.

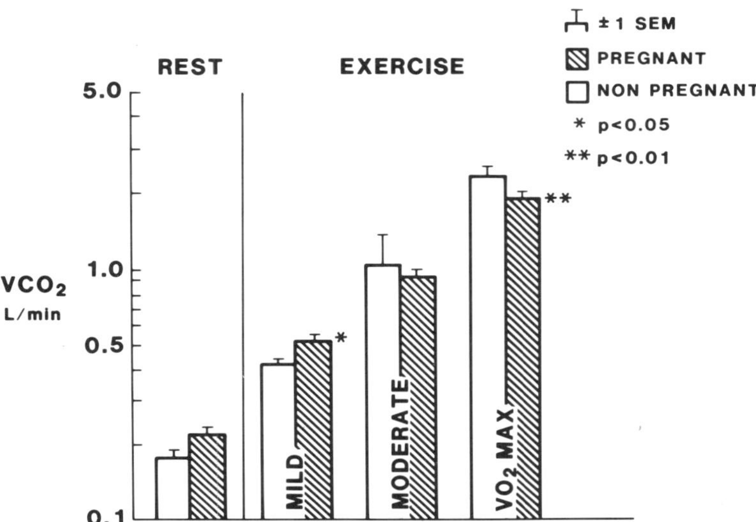

FIGURE 7.4. Carbon dioxide production *(VCO₂)* at rest and as determined at the peak of mild, moderate, and maximal oxygen consumption exercise. (Reprinted with permission from Artal et al, reference 8.)

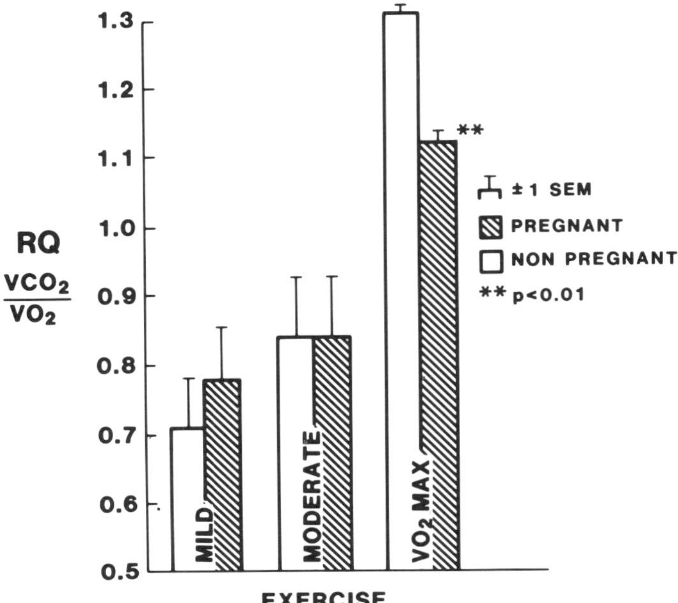

FIGURE 7.5. Respiratory quotient *(RQ)*, or respiratory exchange ratio, at the peak of mild, moderate, and maximal oxygen consumption exercise. (Reprinted with permission from Artal et al, reference 8.)

Fetal Responses to Maternal Exercise

Exercise induces significant hemodynamic shifts, of which the redistribution of blood flow to the exercising muscles away from the visceral organs has the potential to affect the fetus. A reduction in blood flow to the uterus and reduction in gas exchange could potentially lead to maternal respiratory acidosis and fetal hypoxia. In the normal healthy pregnancy, the fetus is affected only rarely during mild and moderate exercise, but the risk increases during strenuous and/or prolonged exercise.

The interactions between fetus and mother compose a fascinating, but often poorly understood, relationship. The fetal well-being and responses to external stimuli could be reflected in fetal behavior, movements, breathing, and heart rates—parameters that have been incorporated into a fetal biophysical profile (9). Recognizing the existence of close correlations between the maternal sympathoadrenal system and fetal behavior, we have studied fetal breathing movements and fetal movement responses to maternal exercise (10) (Figure 7.6).

We have demonstrated a direct relationship between the maternal level

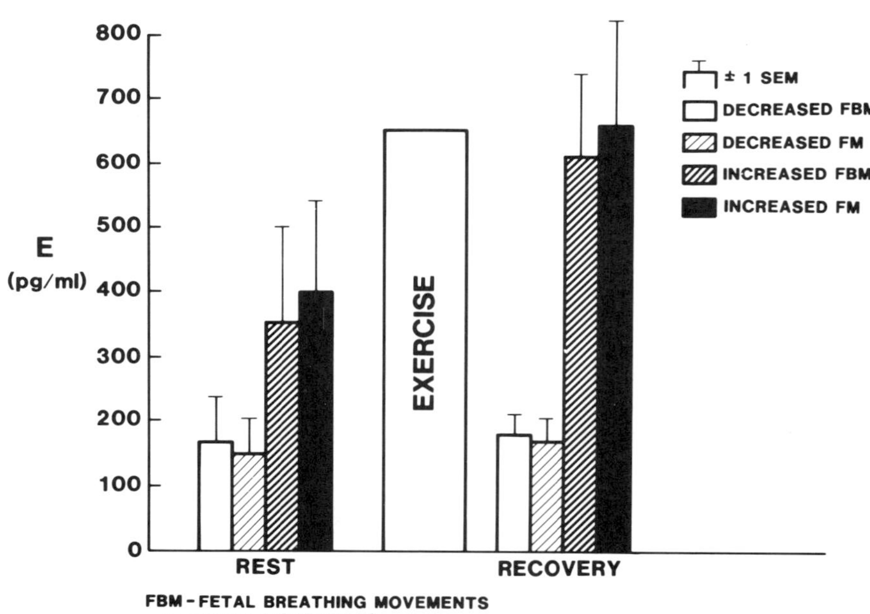

FIGURE 7.6. Fetal breathing movements and fetal movements in relation to maternal plasma epinephrine *(E)* prior to and after exercise. (Reprinted with permission from Platt et al, reference 10.)

of sympathetic activity and the frequency and intensity of fetal response. One could speculate that since the catecholamines modulate plasma glucose levels, fetal activity could be affected. This speculation is supported by strong evidence (11), but is still open to dispute. Among responses, fetal heart rate (FHR) has been studied most extensively. Typical changes in FHR patterns are known to reflect hypoxic and nonhypoxic stress, hypoxia or asphyxia, and sympathetic and parasympathetic activity. Healthy fetuses can tolerate brief periods of hypoxia such as those that may occur during nonstrenuous maternal exercise. By and large, the FHR response to maternal exercise is associated with an increase of approximately 10 to 30 beats per minute (Figure 7.7). Our studies indicate that such changes are consistent and independent of either gestational age (Figure 2, reference 12) or intensity of maternal exercise (12). Nevertheless, in a few isolated cases we have recorded brief episodes of fetal bradycardia in otherwise normal pregnancies (13). We have attributed such events to either temporary fetal cord compression or sustained vagal reflex secondary to major blood volume shifts in both mother and fetus.

Despite the ominous connotations of this event, we hypothesized that such occurrences may be within the realm of normal fetal adaptive responses to major maternal hemodynamic and hormonal shifts. Thus, although apparently well tolerated by normal healthy fetuses, such events may not be tolerated by partially compromised fetuses such as those of diabetic mothers. These findings reinforce the need for medical supervision of exercise programs for special groups of pregnant patients.

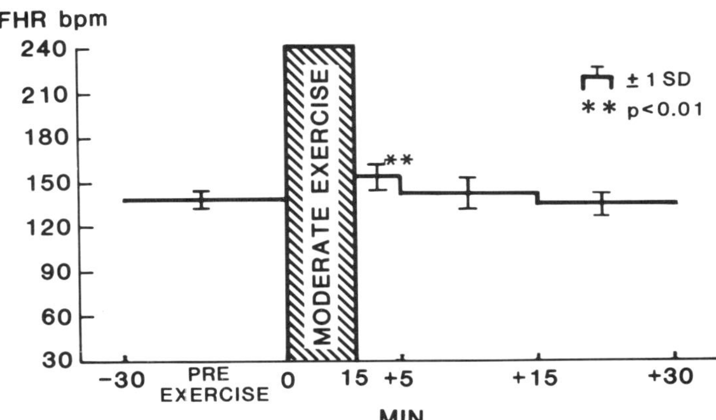

FIGURE 7.7. Fetal heart rate responses to maternal exercise. (Reprinted with permission from Artal et al, reference 12.)

Exercise in the Pregnant Diabetic Woman

Pregnancy should not be a state of confinement, and pregnant diabetic women who had been exercising prior to pregnancy to help maintain normoglycemia may continue to do so in pregnancy, while recognizing that pregnancy brings along a few physiologic limitations. Exercise in pregnancy should be directed towards correcting postural changes, carefully avoiding strain or fatigue, and should be interspersed with periods of rest and relaxation.

Exercise prescription should take into account common orthopedic problems of pregnancy such as those in which edema produces nerve compression syndromes: knee, hip, and back pain; leg cramping; and osteitis pubis. Flexibility and relaxation activities may affect already loose joints and provoke back pain.

Recommendations for exercise in pregnancy should be individualized. Pregnant women should avoid exercise during hot or humid weather, maintain appropriate hydration, stop frequently to rest, eat adequately before exercise, rest afterwards, and be aware of fetal activity. It is important to emphasize that increased uterine activity is a common occurrence after exercise in pregnancy and that in individuals at risk of premature labor, exercise could precipitate undesirable events. Patients should be advised that if uterine contractions become regular and/or occur at intervals of five minutes or less, they should consult their obstetrician. Table 7.1 lists the conditions that contraindicate physical activity during pregnancy.

Pregnant diabetic women could benefit by a balanced therapeutic triad of diet, exercise, and insulin therapy. Exercise for the nonpregnant diabetic woman is usually prescribed at 50% to 70% of her maximal aerobic capacity. As stated, target heart rates for exercise are not available in pregnancy, and owing to wide variations, they will probably never become available. This fact could further complicate exercise prescriptions for the pregnant diabetic woman. Furthermore, one must be aware that the in-

TABLE 7.1. Contraindications for exercise in pregnancy.

Risk of premature labor
Vaginal bleeding during pregnancy
Placenta previa
Anemia
Cardiac disease
Thyroid disease
Hypertension
Intrauterine growth retardation
Malpresentation in the last trimester
Excessive obesity
Extreme underweight

crease in glucose utilization during exercise may lead to hypoglycemia, a major clinical problem in diabetic patients during and after exercise and one with potential adverse effects. For this reason we have conducted studies to evaluate hormonal and metabolic responses to single sessions of mild exercise by comparing normal healthy to uncomplicated diabetic pregnant women. The study was designed to simulate the exercise conditions that may be prescribed for the pregnant diabetic woman (3).

The subject consumed 30 cal/kg ideal body weight, either in the format of an American Diabetes Association diabetic diet or of an equivalent control balanced diet. At the time of testing, mean plasma glucose levels in the diabetic women were 119± 10.5 mg/dL, and each diabetic patient was treated with two daily injections of a mixture of neutral protamine Hagedorn (NPH) insulin and regular insulin. All subjects were placed in a semirecumbent position for a control period of 30 minutes. Maternal heart rate, arterial blood pressure, and FHR were recorded throughout the experiment. Each subject then exercised for a 15-minute period, walking on a motorized treadmill at a constant speed of 2 mph. This type of activity was judged to be light exercise and to generate an approximate energy utilization of 2.33 metabolic equivalents (METs). The oxygen consumption for this type of exercise is estimated to be (0.7 L/min, generating a caloric expenditure (35 cal/min. The exercise was followed by a 30-minute recovery period in a semirecumbent position. Blood samples were collected at 15-minute intervals for selected chemical and hormonal assays.

At present (14) we prescribe a similar, albeit more frequent exercise program for pregnant women with type II diabetes. Patients are asked to use an exercycle at least three days a week, preferably every day, and to exercise 15 minutes after each meal (breakfast, lunch, and dinner) at an intensity of approximately 50% of their maximum aerobic capacity. The subjects are tested in the laboratory once a month after 26 weeks of gestation to determine the maximum aerobic capacity and to adjust the exercise prescription. The subjects are informed of potential complications and are required to keep accurate records of their blood glucose values, which are obtained with home blood glucose monitoring devices. In addition, at approximately 30 weeks, FHR activity is tested weekly by means of a nonstress test and of a log of fetal movements obtained by the patient for one hour after each exercise session. Should any obstetrical or medical complication occur, the patient is instructed to stop the program.

At this time, it is not known if pregnancy is a contributing factor to exercise-related hypoglycemia. Furthermore, most pregnant diabetic patients are unfit and untrained; therefore, they could experience an increased incidence of postexercise hypotension. We believe that the exercise level used in our studies is of adequate intensity to achieve training and to increase glucose utilization. Under the conditions tested, glucose values remained remarkably stable with little variability in either diabetic or nondiabetic pregnant patients. Glucagon levels were not affected by exercise in either group, but were significantly lower in the diabetic patients.

Since epinephrine modulates glucagon release, one could conclude that the epinephrine stimulus generated at this level of exercise was not sufficient to stimulate glucagon release, findings that contrast with our previously published data (7). We speculate that this difference in glucagon and epinephrine response may be due to the slightly higher levels of fitness in our current group of patients. Further evidence that this level of exercise activity is low is that the free fatty acid (FFA) did not change significantly with exercise in either group.

Acute hormone changes are very sensitive to the type, intensity, and duration of exercise. Physical fitness and the basic condition, i.e., fasting or postprandial, are crucial in determining hormonal responses. Insulin modulates glucose uptake by the muscle during exercise. Catecholamines regulate both FFA release by lipolysis and glucose release by means of glycogenolysis. A small increment in epinephrine, as demonstrated in our studies, would facilitate glucose uptake and maintain stable glucose levels. This steady state is essential to the well-being of the fetus. A further surge in epinephrine would inhibit glucose uptake and create a glut of circulating glucose.

Conversely, a significant decrease in plasma glucose can stimulate epinephrine and glucagon release during exercise. In our studies we observed a significant surge in norepinephrine with exercise. Diabetic patients appear to have lower baseline norepinephrine than control subjects, but experience the same absolute increase with exercise. One could speculate that the lower baseline norepinephrine levels are due to a reduced lean body mass in the diabetic patients.

It is important to note that norepinephrine can act as a stimulant to the uterus and may be considered as one of the contributing causes for preterm labor.

We believe that our exercise program is beneficial to pregnant type II diabetic women, possibly by increasing insulin binding and by increasing the postreceptor mechanism of glucose utilization. Although our studies are preliminary, they suggest that the relatively mild aerobic exercise described herein does not have an adverse effect on the pregnant diabetic woman or on her fetus. Whether it is also sufficient to improve glucose tolerance and reduce the need for insulin requirements remains to be determined. Preliminary data indicate that this is the case and suggest that an exercise program should become part of the management of pregnant diabetic women, provided one remembers the potential risks listed in Table 7.2.

In conclusion, we believe that pregnancy should not be a state of confinement and that women should be encouraged to live a normal life and continue their prepregnancy activities, within proper limitations and guidelines.

TABLE 7.2. Risks of exercise in pregnancy.

Maternal
  Musculoskeletal injuries
  Cardiovascular complications
  Premature labor
  Hypoglycemia

Fetal
  Fetal distress
  Intrauterine growth retardation
  Fetal malformations
  Prematurity

References

1. Lawrence RD (1926) The effect of exercise on insulin action in diabetes. Br Med J 1:648–50.
2. Vranic M, Horvath S, Wahren J (1979) Exercise and diabetes: An overview. Diabetes 28(1):107–110.
3. Artal R, Wiswell R, Romem Y (1985) Hormonal responses to exercise in diabetic and nondiabetic pregnant patients. Diabetes 34(2):78–80.
4. Summary and Recommendations of the Second International Workshop Conference on Gestational Diabetes Mellitus (1985) diabetes 34(2):123–126.
5. American College of Obstetricians and Gynecologists (1986) Home exercise programs: Exercise during pregnancy and the postnatal period. Bulletin.
6. Calguneri M, Bird HA, Wright V (1982) Changes in joint laxity occurring during pregnancy. Ann Rheum Dis 41:127.
7. Artal R, Platt DL, Sperling M, Kammula RK, Jilek J, Nakamura R (1981) Exercise in pregnancy. I. Maternal cardiovascular and metabolic responses in normal pregnancy. Am J Obstet Gynecol 140:123–127.
8. Artal R, Wiswell R, Romem Y, Dorey F (1986) Pulmonary responses to exercise in pregnancy. Am J Obstet Gynecol 154:378.
9. Manning FA, Morrison I, Lange IR (1982) Antepartum determination of fetal health: Composite biophysical profile scoring. Clin Perinatol 9:285.
10. Platt LD, Artal R, Semel J, Sipos L, Kammula RK (1983) Exercise in pregnancy. II. Fetal responses. Am J Obstet Gynecol 147:487.
11. Lewis PJ, Trudiuper BJ, Manger J (1979) Effect of maternal glucose on fetal breathing and body movements in late pregnancy. Br J Obstet Gynaecol 85:586.
12. Artal R, Rutherford S, Romem Y, Kammula RK, Dorey FJ, Wiswell RA (1986) Fetal heart rate responses to maternal exercise. Am J Obstet Gynecol 155:729–733.
13. Artal R, Romem Y, Paul RH, Wiswell RA (1984) Fetal bradycardia induced by maternal exercise. Lancet 2:258.
14. Artal R. Unpublished data.

Part IV Obstetrics Management

8
Methods of Fetal Surveillance in Pregnancies Complicated by Diabetes

Luis A. Bracero and Harold Schulman

Introduction

Perinatal mortality in pregnancies complicated by diabetes has decreased dramatically over the years (1–4). To a great extent, this reduction can be attributed to the maintenance of euglycemia (5,6). Of the various factors responsible for the achievement of euglycemia, the most important is the realization that optimal glucose levels in the diabetic pregnant woman are similar to those in the nondiabetic pregnant woman. To maintain these glucose levels, physicians tend to be more liberal with their administration of insulin throughout pregnancy. The advent of self-glucose testing has made it possible to monitor blood sugar levels on a daily basis and to adjust the insulin dosage accordingly.

Some important issues continue to plague the obstetrician caring for pregnant women with diabetes. These issues deal principally with surveillance and, in particular, fetal surveillance. Although infant mortality is no longer a primary problem in the well-controlled diabetic woman, infant morbidity continues to be a concern. Perinatal morbidity in the offspring of a woman with diabetes falls into two categories. One type of morbidity is the result of prematurity and includes the respiratory distress syndrome (RDS), hyperbilirubinemia, and hypocalcemia. The other type is morbidity caused by maternal hyperglycemia and fetal hyperinsulinemia leading to hypoglycemia, macrosomia, erythremia, and multiple congenital anomalies. The morbidity related to prematurity raises another issue: the timing of delivery. If these pregnancies are allowed to go to term, we would, of course, no longer be faced with the problem of prematurity. Instead, the morbidity seen would be that directly associated with glycemic control.

How, then, should one time the delivery in a poorly controlled diabetic gravida, whose offspring, even if at term, may behave much like a premature infant? Clearly, delivering these women early may be compounding the dangers of diabetes with those of prematurity. Thus, the control of maternal blood glucose levels and a close surveillance of the fetus become mandatory.

The mechanism or mechanisms that result in perinatal morbidity and death of the offspring in pregnancies complicated by diabetes are not completely understood. Some studies have suggested that diabetes can lead to placental insufficiency, curtailing the exchange of gases, and ultimately leading to hypoxia and fetal death. Hyperglycemia and fetal hyperinsulinemia appear to be key factors in the pathogenesis of the poor outcome. Shelley's studies on fetal lambs showed that hyperglycemia and mild hypoxemia resulted in acidosis and fetal death (7). Fetuses that were normoglycemic and were made hypoxic and acidotic recovered once the hypoxic insult was removed. Kitzmiller and colleagues' studies on the rhesus monkey also demonstrated that hypoxia in hyperglycemic fetuses leads to severe fetal acidosis (8). Other researchers have documented that fetal hyperinsulinemia leads to fetal hypoxia (9,10).

Maternal assessment of glycemic control includes daily self-monitoring of glucose and monthly determination of glycosylated hemoglobin levels. Fetal surveillance tests are indirect measurements of placental function. These tests include fetal movement counts; estriol (E_3) assays; tests of antepartum fetal heart rate, including nonstress tests (NSTs) and contraction stress tests (CSTs); and fetal biophysical profiles (FBPs). In the following discussion, particular emphasis will be placed upon umbilical artery velocity waveforms (UAVW), a new methodology that promises to identify the fetus who is truly at risk.

Methods of Fetal Surveillance

Fetal Movements

Fetal movement counts have been proposed as a means for assessing fetal well-being (11,12). This test is easily performed by an expectant woman, does not require specialized equipment or laboratory analysis, and involves no cost to the patient. Various methods can be used to perform this test. One of them is the Cardiff "count to ten" system developed by Pearson and Weaver (12) in which the patient is instructed to count the number of fetal movements in a 12-hour period (Figure 8.1). Fewer than ten fetal movements over the given time period have been correlated with impending fetal death. Others (13) propose that after each meal, the woman lie on her left side for 30 minutes and count the number of movements. If fewer than three movements are felt in this time interval, the woman should continue monitoring for another half hour and then up to two hours. If she has still not felt at least 3 movements in one of the half-hour intervals, she should contact her doctor.

Landon and Gabbe used fetal movement counts as the primary means

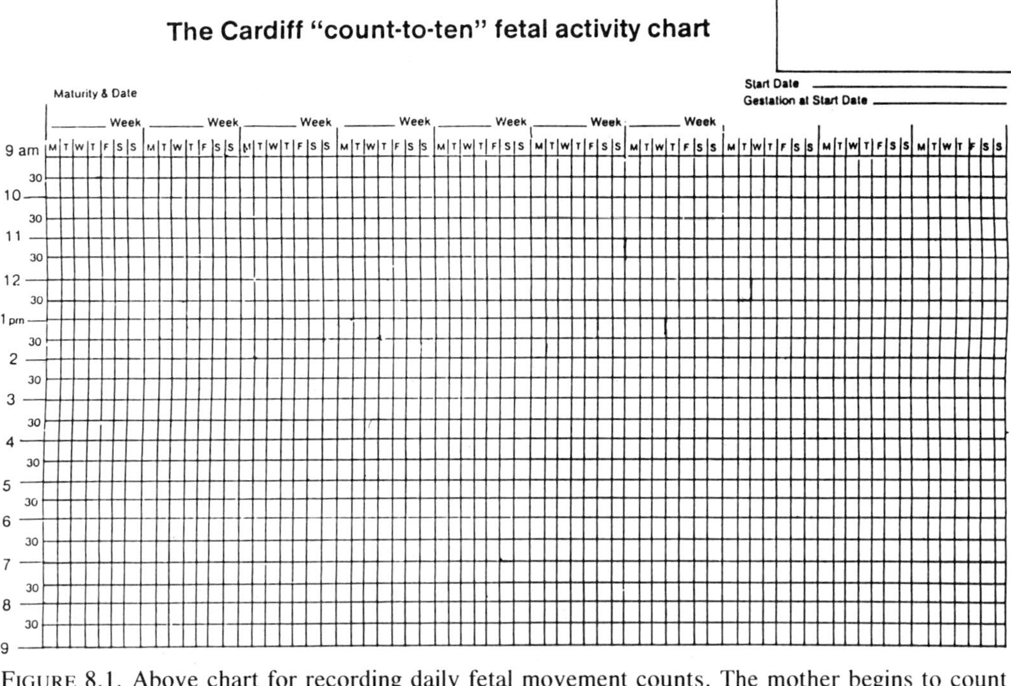

FIGURE 8.1. Above chart for recording daily fetal movement counts. The mother begins to count when she awakes. When ten separate movements have been felt, she marks an X under the appropriate day at the time when the tenth movement is felt. The patient calls the doctor if she has not felt ten movements by 6:00 PM, has not felt the baby move all day, or if it is taking longer to complete the count each day.

of surveillance for their pregnant diabetic population beginning at 28 weeks of gestation (14). No other method of surveillance was instituted until 40 weeks gestation unless other risk factors were ascertained. Weekly NSTs and biweekly urinary E_3 assays were added at 40 weeks or at 34 weeks if risk factors were present. The authors report one patient who had decreased fetal movements at 30 weeks, followed at a later time by a nonreactive NST and a positive CST. She underwent an elective primary cesarean section and was delivered of a healthy baby. The neonatal morbidity rate was about 40% and there were no perinatal deaths.

Stange and colleagues used fetal movement counts as part of a scoring system for the NST in a diabetic population (15). The significance of decreased fetal movements in this population is difficult to assess because the parameters contributing to the score were not individually analyzed, only a total score was given.

Not enough studies have used fetal activity as the primary means of fetal surveillance to provide clinically useful recommendations in pregnancies complicated by diabetes. It might be interesting to see if this type of testing is sufficient to assess fetal well-being.

Estriol Levels

One of the oldest and most widely used methods of assessing fetal health in diabetic pregnant women is the measurement of E_3 levels. This biochemical analysis is performed on a 24-hour urine sample or on plasma. Plasma values are reported as either unconjugated fraction or total E_3.

Estriol measurements must be obtained on a daily basis to be meaningful. Because the 24-hour urine values and total plasma levels tend to fluctuate from day to day, unconjugated E_3 plasma should be obtained. The reported protocols require hospitalization during the third trimester of pregnancy (by 34 weeks gestation) until delivery takes place; otherwise compliance and test accuracy suffer. The majority of investigators perform amniocentesis to establish fetal lung maturity and electively deliver the pregnancies at 38 weeks or earlier. The test is considered positive if there is a significant drop in the E_3 level compared with the mean value of the previous three days. The definition of a significant drop varies; it is a 35% decrease for some, a 40% or 50% decrease for others. Unfortunately, the percentage of false positives is high.

Some investigators have studied the effectiveness of E_3 levels in predicting fetal distress or well-being in pregnancies complicated by diabetes. Whittle and associates used unconjugated daily plasma E_3 as the primary tool for fetal surveillance, with antepartum fetal heart rate testing (AFHRT) as backup in 70 insulin-dependent diabetic patients (16). Ten percent of these pregnancies were terminated electively prior to 38 weeks owing to presumed or documented fetal distress. The rate of cesarean delivery was much higher in patients electively delivered than in those who went into spontaneous labor (60% v 25%). The authors conclude that daily E_3 measurements constitute a valuable test for assessing fetal status. However, recognizing the significant rate of false positive results, they recommend that the test be used in conjunction with other tests. Jorge et al (17) confirmed that false positive results could be eliminated by using E_3 measurements in combination with AFHRT. They conclude that the major benefit of this combination of tests is in determining when not to intervene. Strange et al published a retrospective study comparing 24-hour urinary E_3 excretion and daily NSTs in 76 diabetic women during the last trimester of pregnancy (15). Two neonatal deaths were reported and attributed to congenital anomalies; neither of these cases demonstrated abnormal E_3 values or abnormal NSTs. Seven newborns showed signs of asphyxia (Apgar score <7). Forty two women had a drop in E_3 levels of 30% to 50%, leading the authors to conclude that a large number of these patients did not have placental insufficiency. Even an E_3 drop of more than 50% could be a false positive sign. On the other hand, more than one abnormal NST was always predictive of fetal distress. The authors believe that daily NSTs should replace E_3 determinations, thereby eliminating many unnecessary premature interventions. Ray et al followed 107 insulin-dependent pregnant women by means of serum unconjugated E_3 levels and CSTs (18). In the group of patients who showed at least one significant decrease in E_3 levels, there were no more positive CSTs than in the group without any decrease. Also, there was no statistical difference in perinatal outcome. The authors state that a significant drop in E_3 values should never be used as the sole determinant for intervention and that, in addition, the test is expensive and time consuming for the patient. They also felt that the results do not add decisive information about fetal distress even if used in conjunction with fetal heart rate stress testing. Therefore, the authors cannot justify continued use of E_3 measurements. Based on the available data, we agree with the authors that the time has come to stop using E_3 values for monitoring pregnancies complicated by diabetes.

Antepartum Fetal Heart Rate Testing

As stated above, fetal heart rate monitoring has been used in conjunction with E_3 for fetal surveillance. There are two types of fetal heart rate tests, the NST and the CST (Figure 8.2). The NST basically measures the integrity of the fetal central nervous system, and the CST attempts to measure the fetal response to diminished transport. The methodology for performing both of these tests has been extensively described (19,20).

A few investigators have advocated AFHRT as the primary method of fetal surveillance in diabetic women. Miller and Horger performed a retrospective study on 54 pregnant women with insulin-dependent diabetes who had an AFHRT within seven days of delivery or in whom there were fetal deaths (21). Nonstress tests had been obtained weekly starting at 28

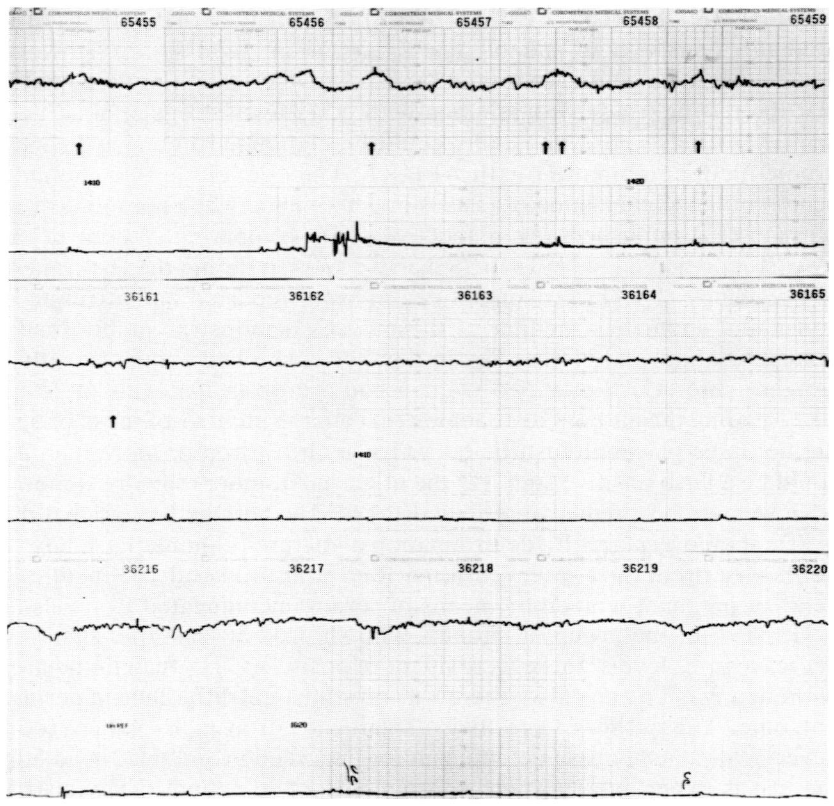

FIGURE 8.2. The top tracing shows a reactive NST that indicates fetal well-being. The middle tracing is a non reactive NST and the bottom tracing is a positive CST; both of these tracings are suggestive of fetal distress.

to 34 weeks gestation, depending on the patient's clinical condition, and the patients with normal AFHRT had been allowed to go to term. If the NST was nonreactive it was followed by a CST. If the CST was negative, the patient was retested one week later; if the CST was positive, the patient was delivered. There were four cases of fetal death, one of which was a set of twins, and all had occurred four to seven days after a reactive NST or a negative CST. All three mothers had suboptimal glycemic control. The authors state that NSTs and CSTs have the same predictive value and advocate the use of NSTs for initial screening. Because all of the fetal deaths occurred within four to seven days after normal test results, they conclude that fetal heart rate testing should be performed at least biweekly. Diamond et al reported on 119 insulin-dependent patients followed primarily with NSTs beginning at 32 weeks gestation (22). If the NST was reactive, it was repeated biweekly; if nonreactive, it was followed immediately by a CST. If the CST was negative, biweekly NSTs were resumed; if positive, delivery was carried out. There was one intrauterine fetal death attributed to maternal diabetic ketoacidosis. Fourteen women had nonreactive NSTs followed by positive CSTs. Six infants had major congenital anomalies; the other eight infants were delivered without confirmatory evidence of fetal distress (Apgar Scores >7). In addition, there were two neonatal deaths associated with heart abnormalities. One was preceded by a nonreactive NST and a negative CST; the other had a reactive NST. The authors conclude that early delivery in women with abnormal AFHRT prevented unexplained stillbirths. However, they did not explore the significance of false positive results. Teramo et al used the NST in 145 insulin-dependent women (23). Testing was begun at 32 weeks gestation and was performed every other day until the 34th week of gestation and daily thereafter. All patients were hospitalized by the 32nd week of gestation. Contraction stress testing was not used following a nonreactive NST. In the event of an abnormal NST, delivery took place. No fetal deaths were reported. Patients were divided according to the results of fetal heart rate testing, and a retrospective analysis of diabetic control was performed. The authors found that the majority of patients with abnormal NSTs had elevated glycosylated hemoglobin levels, which implies poor glycemic control. Few patients with optimal glycemic control had abnormal NSTs. The authors expressed a concern with sudden fetal demise and, therefore, they recommend that NSTs be performed daily or every other day.

Thus, the recommended frequency of fetal heart rate testing and the time when they are to start varies with individual protocols. Nevertheless, it is clear that poor glucose regulation leads to abnormal heart rate tests and poor pregnancy outcome. The NST lends itself for outpatient monitoring because it is quick and easy to perform. This ease of monitoring reduces the need to hospitalize the diabetic woman who is in good glycemic control and has no other complications. However, many physicians still feel more comfortable hospitalizing the diabetic woman. It can be deduced from the above studies that the diabetic woman in good control does not need daily NSTs to provide reassurance of fetal well-being. On the other hand, the woman with poor glycemic control is at high risk of fetal death and should be monitored more closely; the optimal interval remains to be determined.

Fetal Biophysical Profile

The FBP has been proposed as the primary method of fetal surveillance (24) or as an alternative to the CST following a nonreactive NST (25). This test can be beneficial in patients where the CST is contraindicated, such as those with previous cesarean sections, placenta previa, premature rupture of membranes, or at risk of premature labor. A fetal biophysical profile involves five parameters: fetal breathing movements, fetal tone, gross fetal body movements, amniotic fluid volume, and fetal heart rate. All of these variables, except for the fetal heart rate, are assessed by means of a real-time ultrasound examination. Each variable is scored independently; two points are given if a parameter is normal, and zero points if abnormal (Table 8.1). A total score of 8 to 10 points is considered an indication of fetal well-being. The significance of a score of 4 to 6 is uncertain and an indication that the tests should be repeated in 24 hours or that the patient should be delivered. A score of 0 to 2 is indicative of fetal jeopardy and commands immediate intervention.

Only one study reports the use of this test in the management of diabetic pregnancies. Golde and associates (26) performed NSTs twice weekly starting at 34 weeks gestation in 107 insulin-dependent gravidas. When the NST was nonreactive, the other four parameters of FBP were evaluated. A score of 8 was considered evidence of fetal well-being. A score of less than 8 was followed with either a CST or a repeat FBP. Additionally, 85 of these patients had serial FBP despite reactive NSTs and in 99% of them the score was 8 to 10. The authors concluded that a score of 8 on an FBP following a nonreactive NST provides assurance that the fetus is

TABLE 8.1. The fetal biophysical profile scoring system.

Parameter	0 Point	2 Points	Score given
Fetal breathing	The absence of breathing movement or an episode of breathing movement of less than 30 seconds' duration during a 30-minute period.	Minimum one episode of fetal breathing of 30 seconds' duration in a 30-minute observation period.	
Fetal tone	Extremities extended Spine extended Fetal hand open Movement not followed by flexion	Extremities flexed Trunk flexed Head flexed on chest Movement followed by flexion	
Fetal movement	Two or less discrete fetal movements in 30 minutes	Minimum of three discrete fetal movements in 30 minutes	
Amniotic fluid volume	Fluid absent in most areas of uterine cavity Pockets seen measure 2 cm or less on vertical axis Crowding of fetal small parts	Fluid evident throughout Pockets of fluid measure more than 2 cm on vertical diameter	
NST	One or no accelerations in 40 minutes	Two or more accelerations in 20 minutes	
		Total	

Adapted from Manning et al (27).

not in trouble. On the other hand, they recommend that a diabetic woman with a score of less than 8 be evaluated further by a CST.

Umbilical Artery Velocity Waveforms

A new placental function test is the UAVW. This test measures the resistance to umbilical artery flow velocity by the placenta. The amount of resistance is determined by calculating a systolic to diastolic ratio from the velocity waveform. A continuous Doppler ultrasound with a 4-MHz transducer, a power density of 6.5 mW/cm^2, and a spectrum analyzer has been used to identify and measure the velocity of the red blood cells as they move through the umbilical artery. The methodology for recording velocity waveforms is simple. A Doppler probe is placed on the pregnant woman's abdomen as she lies in a slightly tilted supine position. Four fetal signals can be identified. The cardiac signal has small valvular oscillations and scattered echoes; the aortic signal is characterized by a sharp rise and fall, appears triangular, and has a ratio of 7 or 8 to 1; the umbilical vein signal has a nonpulsating flow pattern; and the umbilical artery signal is triangular with a tapering diastolic component. A real-time sonogram is used to localize the umbilical cord when the UAVW signal is not readily identified. The image obtained is freeze-framed, and a cursor is used to measure the systolic (S) peak and the diastolic (D) trough. A ratio is then calculated (Figure 8.3). During each examination four separate fields of waveforms are analyzed and the mean S/D ratio is recorded.

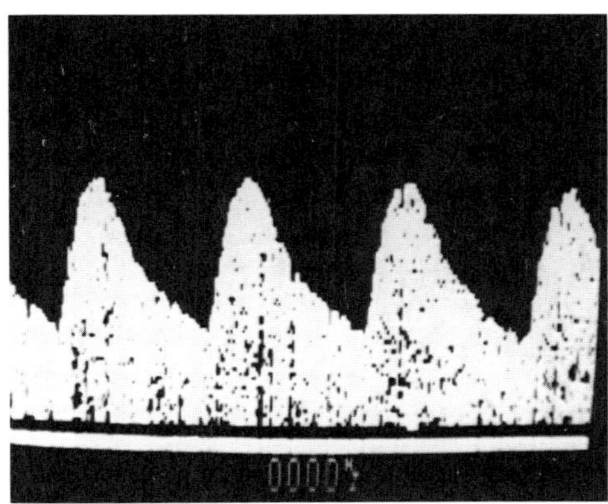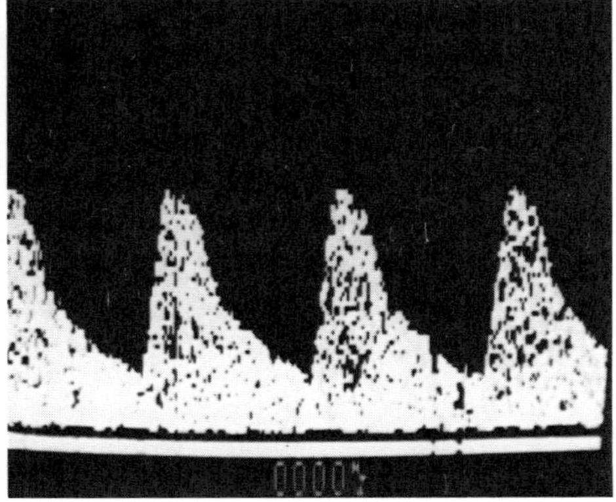

FIGURE 8.3. Normal and abnormal umbilical artery velocity waveforms are illustrated. On the left the S/D ratio is 2:2 (normal) and on the right the S/D ratio is 3:4 (abnormal). (From Bracero et al (1986). Obstetrics and Gynecology 68:654–658. Reprinted with permission from The American College of Obstetricians and Gynecologists.)

We have performed 140 UAVW examinations in 43 pregnant diabetic women, 25 of whom were insulin-dependent (28). These examinations were carried out at the time of scheduled prenatal visits during the third trimester of pregnancy. When the patient population was divided into a good and a poor glycemic-control group, a significant difference in the S/D ratio was observed. The group of women with poor control, defined as a mean third-trimester glucose value of 120 mg/dL or more, had a mean SD ratio greater than 3. Schulman et al (29) reported that an S/D ratio of less than 3 during the third trimester is indicative of normal placental vascular resistance. Therefore, an S/D ratio equal to or greater than 3 implies increased placental vascular resistance. A linear relationship between third-trimester S/D ratios and mean blood glucose is seen in Figure 8.4. It will be observed that the majority of patients with elevated blood glucose levels had increased placental vascular resistance. We concluded from the data that maternal hyperglycemia leads to placental vascular disease, which is believed to be the cause of increased perinatal morbidity and mortality

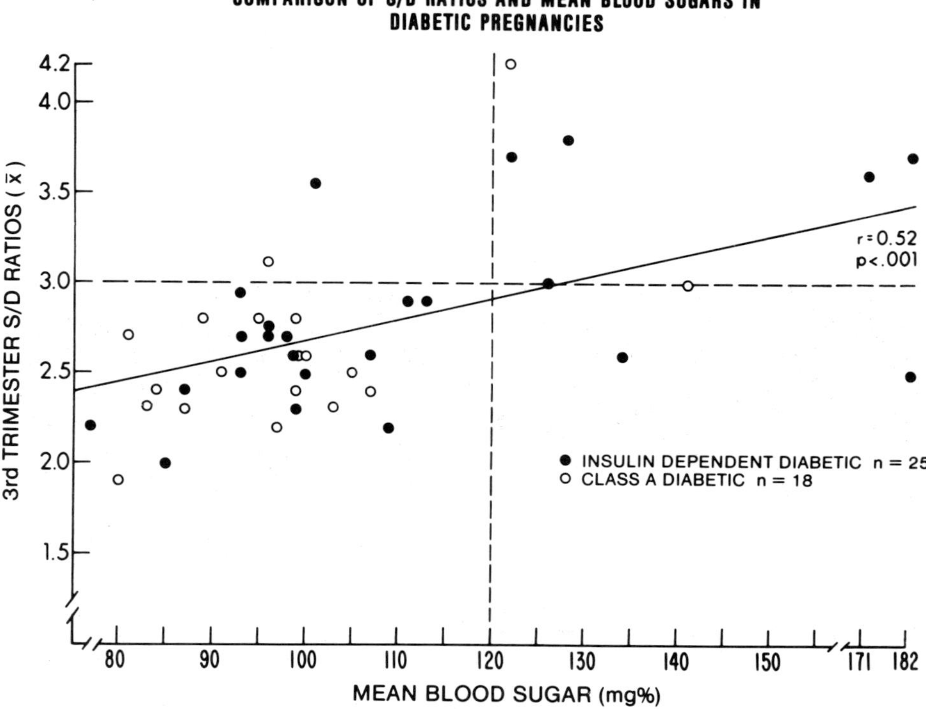

FIGURE 8.4. Scatter diagram showing the relationship between umbilical artery S/D ratios and mean blood sugar values during the third trimester. A linear regression analysis reveals a positive correlation. (From Bracero et al (1986). Obstetrics and Gynecology 68:654–658. Reprinted with permission from The American College of Obstetricians and Gynecologists.)

TABLE 8.2. Predictive value of abnormal blood glucose levels in identifying increased placental vascular resistance.

| | No. of cases | | |
	Positive test	Negative test	
Increased vascular resistance	7	2	78% Sensitivity
Normal vascular resistance	2	32	94% Specificity

Positive test = mean blood glucose ⩾ 120 mg/dL; increased vascular resistance = Average S/D Ratio ⩾ 3; predictive value of a positive test = 78%; predictive value of a negative test = 94%.

seen in the pregnancies of diabetic women. Indeed, the poorly controlled group had a significantly higher incidence of antepartum mortality and neonatal morbidity.

The predictive value of poor blood glucose regulation in identifying increased placental vascular resistance can be calculated from the data (Table 8.2). It will be noted that in seven out of nine patients with increased placental vascular resistance and in two out of 34 patients with normal placental vascular resistance, the mean blood glucose was equal to or greater than 120 mg/dL. The sensitivity for the detection of increased placental vascular resistance is 78% and the specificity is 94%. The predictive value of a normal mean blood glucose in identifying the absence of disease is 94%. These data indicate that glycemic control influences placental vascular resistance and that increased placental vascular resistance, as determined by elevated UAVW S/D ratios, is associated with poor glycemic control and poor outcome in pregnancies complicated by diabetes.

We have continued to study UAVWs and their usefulness in evaluating the placental function in diabetes and pregnancy and have found that in a diabetic population with good glycemic control, the majority of UAVWs are normal and are associated with reactive NSTs and good pregnancy outcomes. In a single patient with relatively good glycemic control (mean glucose 110 mg/dL) and an S/D ratio greater than 3 (S/D ratio = 3.8), the NST was abnormal. She was delivered by primary cesarean section owing to fetal distress; the newborn was small for gestational age and required phototherapy for hyperbilirubinemia. Normal UAVWs provided reassurance that the fetuses were healthy during the last trimester and minimized unnecessary intervention.

Conclusion

We conclude that the UAVW provides an important additional mode of surveillance for pregnancies associated with diabetes. Theoretically it tests placental vascular integrity more directly than the other tests that we have described. This test is unique because placental disease is probably the major cause of the perinatal morbidity and mortality seen in a pregnant woman with diabetes. The patient does not need to be hospitalized to have this test performed, nor does UAVW need be performed as frequently as other tests, yet it may be more predictive of pregnancy outcome than the other tests described.

We recommend that the patient with good glycemic control and a normal UAVW during the third trimester be followed with weekly NSTs to reassure the physician and the mother that the fetus is healthy. Velocity waveforms should be performed early in the third trimester (28 weeks gestation) and bimonthly thereafter. The NSTs should be initiated at 34 weeks. Additionally, daily fetal movement counts are a good indicator of fetal health and should be encouraged during the third trimester. A real-time sonogram should be performed at 38 weeks gestation to assess the pregnancy and, in particular, the fetal weight and the amount of amniotic fluid. It has become increasingly clear that some of the morbidity seen in pregnancies with diabetes is due to premature delivery. Therefore, all efforts should be made to carry the pregnancies of well-controlled diabetic women with normal S/D ratios to term. The poorly controlled diabetic gravida is very likely to have an abnormal UAVW S/D ratio. She should be hospitalized promptly to try to achieve better glycemic control. An abnormal S/D ratio places the pregnancy at higher risk. Whether fetal surveillance of pregnancies with high S/D ratios is safe in a hospital setting remains to be determined. Until further data are available, it is probably safer to deliver the pregnancies with poor glycemic control and an abnormal S/D ratio. If one wished to delay the delivery, the pregnancy could be followed with weekly UAVW, daily fetal movement counts, and biweekly NSTs to ascertain trends.

The ultimate goal is to delay the time of delivery as long as possible, ideally, until spontaneous labor occurs, unless other pregnancy complications develop.

References

1. Gugliucci CL, O'Sullivan MJ, Opperman W, et al (1976) Intensive care of the pregnant diabetic. Am J Obstet Gynecol 125:435–441.
2. Gyves MT, Rodman HM, Little AB, et al (1977) A modern approach to management of pregnant diabetics: A two year analysis of outcomes. Am J Obstet Gynecol 128:606–616.
3. Kitzmiller JL, Cloherty JP, Younger DM, et al (1978) Diabetic pregnancy and perinatal morbidity. Am J Obstet Gynecol 131:560–580.
4. Coustan DR, Berkowitz RL, Hobbins JC (1980) Tight metabolic control of overt diabetes in pregnancy. Am J Med 68:845–852.
5. Adashi EY, Pinto H, and Tyson JE (1979) Impact of maternal euglycemia on fetal outcome in diabetic pregnancy. Am J Obstet Gynecol 133:268–274.

6. Jovanovic L, Druzin M, Peterson CM (1981) Effect of euglycemia on the outcome of pregnancy in insulin dependent diabetic women as compared with normal control subjects. Am J Med 71:921–927.
7. Shelley HJ (1973) The use of chronically catheterized foetal lambs for the study of foetal metabolism, in Comline KS, Cross KW, Dawes GS, Nathanielsz PW (eds): Foetal and Neonatal Physiology. Cambridge University Press, London pp 360–381.
8. Kitzmiller JL, Phillippe M, Von Oeyen P, et al (1981) Hyperglycemia, hypoxia, and fetal acidosis in rhesus monkeys. Abstract Proceedings of the 28th Annual Meeting Society for Gynecological Investigation.
9. Carson BS, Phillipps AF, Simmons MA, et al (1980) Effects of sustained insulin infusion upon glucose uptake and oxygenation of the ovine fetus. Pediatr Res 14:147–152.
10. Quisell BJ, Bonds DR, Krell BS, et al (1980) The effects of chronic fetal insulin infusions upon fetal oxygenation. Clin Res 28:125A.
11. Sadovsky E, Yaffe H (1973) Daily fetal movement recording and fetal prognosis. Obstet Gynecol 41:845–850.
12. Pearson JF, Weaver JB (1976) Fetal activity and fetal wellbeing: an evaluation. Br Med J 1:1305–1307.
13. Goldberg JD, Jornsay DL, Hausknecht RU (1985) Diabetes in pregnancy, in Cherry SH, Berkowitz RL, Kase NG (eds): Rovinsky and Guttmacher's Medical, Surgical, and Gynecologic Complications of Pregnancy. Williams & Wilkins, Baltimore, pp 408–419.
14. Landon MB, Gabbe SG (1985) Antepartum fetal surveillance in gestational diabetes mellitus. Diabetes 34:50–54.
15. Stange L, Stangeberg M, Carlstrom K, et al (1985) Surveillance of the diabetic pregnancy with antepartum fetal nonstress testing and urinary estriol excretion. Gynecol Obstet Invest 20:141–148.
16. Whittle MJ, Anderson D, Lowensohn RI, et al (1979) VI. Experience with unconjugated plasma estriol assays and antepartum fetal heart rate testing in diabetic pregnancies. Am J Obstet Gynecol 135:764–772.
17. Jorge CS, Artal R, Paul RH, et al (1981) Antepartum fetal surveillance in diabetic pregnant patients. Am J Obstet Gynecol 141:641–645.
18. Ray DA, Yeast JD, Freeman RK (1986) The current role of daily serum estriol monitoring in the insulin dependent pregnant diabetic woman. Am J Obstet Gynecol 154:1257–1263.
19. Freeman RK (1975) The use of the oxytocin challenge test for antepartum clinical evaluation of uteroplacental respiratory function. Am J Obstet Gynecol 121:481–489.
20. Everston LR, Gauthier RJ, Schifrin BS, et al (1979) Antepartum fetal heart rate testing I Evolution of the nonstress test. Am J Obstet Gynecol 133:29–33.
21. Miller JM, Horger EO (1985) Antepartum heart rate testing in diabetic pregnancy. J Reprod Med 30:515–517.
22. Diamond MP, Vaughn WK, Salyer SL, et al (1985) Antepartum fetal monitoring in insulin dependent diabetic pregnancies. Am J Obstet Gynecol 153:528–533.
23. Teramo K, Ammala P, Ylinen K, et al (1983) Pathologic fetal heart rate associated with poor metabolic control in diabetic pregnancies. Obstet Gynecol 61:559–565.

24. Manning FA, Lange IR, Morrison I, et al (1984) Fetal biophysical profile score and the nonstress test: A comparative trial. Obstet Gynecol 64:326–331.
25. Vintzileos AM, Campbell WA, Ingardia CJ, et al (1983) The fetal biophysical profile and its predictive value. Obstet Gynecol 62:271–278.
26. Golde SH, Montoro M, Good-Anderson B, et al (1984) The role of nonstress tests, fetal biophysical profile, and contraction stress tests in an outpatient management of insulin requiring diabetic pregnancies. Am J Obstet Gynecol 148:269–273.
27. Manning FA, Morrison I, Lange IR, et al (1982) Antepartum determination of fetal health: Composite biophysical profile scoring. Clin Perinatol 9:285–296.
28. Bracero L, Schulman H, Fleischer A, et al (1986) Umbilical artery velocimetry in diabetes and pregnancy. Obstet Gynecol. 68:654–658.
29. Schulman H, Fleischer A, Stern W, et al (1984) Umbilical velocity wave ratios in human pregnancies. Am J Obstet Gynecol 148:985–990.

9
Diabetes in Pregnancy: Considerations for the Management of Delivery

M.I. DRURY

Introduction

Throughout normal pregnancy, metabolic adaptations occur so that a constant fuel supply may be provided for the life and development of the fetus. These adaptations begin quite early when, in response to rising levels of estrogen and progesterone in the mother, the fetal β-cells become hyperplastic and secrete more insulin, which, in turn, results in greater utilization of glucose, increased glycogen storage, and a reduction in the output of glucose from the liver; in other words, an anabolic state is created. The simplest evidence of this change is a reduction in the maternal fasting blood glucose level. Maternal or exogenous insulin does not cross the placenta, and the fetus secretes insulin from its own β-cells from the eighth week of gestation (1). Glucose is transferred across the placenta by facilitated diffusion, while amino acids (alanine being the most important because it stimulates the fetal β-cells) are actively transported by the placenta to the fetus. Consequently, the activity of fetal β-cells is determined by the maternal blood glucose and amino acid levels. "Giant" islets are a common finding at autopsy in infants of diabetic mothers in whom diabetic control has been inadequate.

As pregnancy advances, the metabolic adaptations intensify, with the primary aim of providing a constant supply of nutrients to the fetus. These adaptations are mediated through increasing maternal levels of estrogens, progesterone, prolactin, free cortisol, and placental lactogen, which lead to a progressive increase in tissue resistance to insulin at a postreceptor site. In turn, the increased resistance is counterbalanced by increased secretion of insulin by the maternal β-cells.

As Freinkel has shown, these changes are designed to provide nutrients to the fetus at all times. Thus, when the mother is fasting, her metabolic state is one of "accelerated starvation," and when she is feeding, it is one of "facilitated anabolism" (2). The state of "accelerated starvation" provides the setting in which ketoacidosis may occur.

In summary, the metabolic adaptations of pregnancy result in a lowering of the fasting blood glucose level and an increasing output of insulin, the latter being particularly marked during the last 20 weeks. In discussing diabetes mellitus in pregnancy, and in light of the above information, the following practical points are considered:

1. As pregnancy advances, some previously healthy patients develop gestational diabetes mellitus (GDM).
2. The standard criteria for the diagnosis of diabetes mellitus are not applicable in pregnancy.
3. There is an increase in insulin requirement as pregnancy advances.
4. The criteria of strict metabolic control are different during pregnancy.

Gestational Diabetes Mellitus

As pregnancy advances, the increasing tissue resistance to insulin creates a demand for more insulin. In the great majority of women, this demand can readily be supplied by their β-cells so that the balance between resistance to insulin and available insulin is maintained. If, however, β-cell reserve is impaired, insulin resistance becomes dominant and hyperglycemia develops. Depending on the degree of insulin deficiency, hyperglycemia may be mild and difficult to detect but easy to control by dietary restriction, or it may be florid and require exogenous insulin. Whether the carbohydrate intolerance is mild or severe, it is important that it be detected because when unrecognized, it is associated with significant perinatal mortality.

In the majority of such cases the carbohydrate intolerance develops in the last half (especially the last 6 weeks) of pregnancy, at which time insulin resistance increases progressively until delivery when, in most cases, it rapidly disappears. In a minority of cases the insulin resistance persists after the puerperium—more probably in women in whom hyperglycemia had developed in early pregnancy. This phenomenon is understandable when one realizes that if hyperglycemia develops before there has been a marked increase in insulin resistance, significant impairment of β-cell reserve is likely to be present.

Detection of Gestational Diabetes

Clues that suggest the presence of GDM are:

• family history of diabetes, especially in first-degree relatives;
• glucose in a "second fasting" urine sample (see below);
• a history of unexplained perinatal loss;
• a history of a "large for gestational age" infant;
• a history of a malformed infant;
• gross maternal obesity (200 lb or more).

Other pointers, perhaps of lesser significance, include parity greater than 5, recurrent toxemia of pregnancy, and recurrent premature labor. The presence of more than one clue increases the likelihood that disordered carbohydrate tolerance exists.

Glycosuria is a common finding in pregnancy since in about 15% of pregnant women, there is a temporary lowering of the renal threshold for glucose. Thus, investigations based on glycosuria alone would not be fruitful. However, the specificity of the finding can be increased if one uses the presence of glucose in a "second fasting" urine specimen on two occasions as an index of suspicion. The urine voided on waking is dis-carded and a fresh specimen is passed about 15 minutes later while the woman is still fasting. This latter test reflects the FBG, which in a normal pregnant woman, is not likely to exceed even a low renal threshold. Suspect cases should be seen fortnightly for the usual antenatal measurements, with special emphasis on weight control. The postprandial blood glucose is measured at each visit, and if it does not exceed 6.5 mmol/L (117 mg/dL), an oral glucose tolerance test (OGTT) is deferred until the 37th or 38th week of gestation, when the demand upon the islets is maximal. If, at any visit, the postprandial blood glucose exceeds 6.5 mmol/L, an OGTT is done immediately. Should the test be positive, the diagnosis of abnormal carbohydrate tolerance of pregnancy can be made. A normal OGTT at an early stage of pregnancy does *not*, however, exclude the diagnosis and the test must be repeated at 37 or 38 weeks before a definitive decision is made. Patients who have a negative OGTT at 37 or 38 weeks are treated as normal patients. If the OGTT is positive, the patient is placed on a diet and observed in the same way as any diabetic woman. If the criteria of ideal control (see above) are not rapidly achieved, insulin is introduced. In well-controlled, uncomplicated cases, the pregnancy is allowed to continue until spontaneous labor occurs.

A high insulin requirement does not necessarily mean that the diabetic state will persist after delivery. We have had many patients who required 40 to 60 units daily during pregnancy and in whom the OGTT became normal during the puerperium (Tables 9.1 and 9.2).

TABLE 9.1. Gestational diabetes mellitus requiring insulin during pregnancy.

Maturity (wks)		Postprandial blood glucose	
		(mmol/L)	(mg/dL)
17		5.8	104
20		13.2	238
		14.0	252
27	Insulin dosage	8.1	146
33	increased to	5.8	104
38	60 U/d	5.9	90

The oral glucose tolerance test was normal after the puerperium.

TABLE 9.2. Evolution from GDM to clinical DM.

B.K.	A45333	b. 1951	No FH of DM
1979	0^{+0}	OGTT at 36 weeks for glycosuria	
		4.3 - 6.5- 9.3 - *10.5* - *10.8* mmol/L	
		(77, 117, 167, 189, 194 mg/dL)	
		After the puerperium	
		3.7 - 7.8 - 7.8 - 8.5 - 8.0	
		(67, 140, 140, 153, 144 mg/dL)	
1980	1^{+0}	OGTT at 16 weeks:	
		5.6 - 12 - 14.7 - 14 mmol/L	
		(101, 216, 265, 252 mg/dL)	
		R_x Insulin 24 units daily	
		After the puerperium:	
		10.8 - 18.3 - 20.2 - 22.8 - 22 mmol/L	
		(194, 329, 364, 410, 396 mg/dL)	

B.K., patient's initials; A45333, hospital chart numbers; b., born; FH, family history; DM, diabetes mellitus.

Follow-Up of Women With GDM

After the puerperium the OGTT is repeated, and if found positive, the diagnosis is changed from GDM to clinical diabetes mellitus, that is, diabetes that happened to manifest itself for the first time during pregnancy.

As some patients with GDM develop clinical diabetes later in life, they should be advised to maintain a normal body weight, informed about the significance of polydipsia and polyuria, and encouraged to seek annual examinations and to return immediately should they again conceive.

In any unexplained stillbirth, the possibility of gestational diabetes should be considered, and at autopsy special attention should be paid to the histology of the pancreas and gonads. Islet cell hyperplasia (in the absence of an ABO-Rh blood group incompatibility problem), increased interstitial tissue in the testis, or luteinization of the theca interna of the ovary is indicative of maternal diabetes even if the OGTT is normal, since glucose intolerance rapidly disappears after delivery. Glycosylated hemoglobin measurements rarely help because the degree of hyperglycemia is usually insufficient to cause an abnormal degree of glycosylation. These women require special supervision during subsequent pregnancies.

Criteria for the Diagnosis of Diabetes During Pregnancy

In a normal pregnancy, fasting and postprandial blood glucose levels are respectively lower and higher than in the nonpregnant state; i.e., the peaks are higher and the valleys are lower. For these reasons, the standard criteria for diagnosis of diabetes mellitus cannot be applied during pregnancy. In spite of this, the Expert Committee of the World Health Organization (WHO) recommended that the criteria for diagnosing "diabetes in pregnancy" should be the same as those used in nonpregnant adults (3). The National Diabetes Data Group (NDDG) does not share this view (4), nor do I. Instead, following the recommendation of O'Sullivan and Mahan (5), I base the diagnosis on the results of a three-hour, 100-g OGTT. With this test, the upper limits of normal are as follows: fasting plasma, 5.8 mmol/L (105 mg/dL); one plasma hour, 10.6 mmol/L (190 mg/dL); two plasma hours, 9.2 mmoL/L (165 mg/dL); three plasma hours, 8.1 mmoL/L (145 mg/dL). If any two of these values are equalled or exceeded, the test is positive. It should be noted that when the OGTT is performed *after the puerperium*, standard methodology (75 g glucose) and criteria (fasting >140 mg/dL and two-hour value >200 mg/dL) then apply.

Effect of Pregnancy on Insulin Requirements

In the second half of pregnancy the normal hormonal changes create a degree of insulin resistance that is overcome by an increased insulin output. The counterpart of this in women with insulin-dependent diabetes is a gradual increase in insulin requirement as pregnancy progresses.

Alteration in Standards of Control

In normal pregnancy FBG levels are lower (4 rather than 5 mmol/L, or 72 rather than 90 mg/dL) and postprandial levels are higher (7 rather than 6.5 mmol/L or 126 rather than 117 mg/dL) than in the nonpregnant state. These are the values by which metabolic control during pregnancy should be evaluated.

Significance of Gestational Diabetes

Jarrett (6) maintains that "there seems no reason to believe that haphazard screening for GDM has contributed in any way to the overall reduction in perinatal mortality rates," and after studying the literature he concluded that "the obsession with BG (or glucose tolerance) has led to a neglect of other factors which may be much more important in determining or predicting fetal survival." Furthermore, he argues that "it is impossible from the data available to determine whether the risk is directly attributable to hyperglycemia or whether hyperglycemia or impaired glucose tolerance is a marker for one or more factors which are truly causal."

It may be true that *haphazard* screening for GDM is unrewarding, but that does not mean that *selective screening* is. Conceding that screening based on specific clues (see above) will uncover more chaff than wheat, the reward may still be worthwhile because unrecognized carbohydrate intolerance during pregnancy—whether due to GDM or pregestational (clinical) diabetes mellitus—is, in our experience, associated with perinatal loss.

Clinical Diabetes and Pregnancy

In the preinsulin era, pregnancy in the diabetic woman was rare and dangerous. Almost certainly, only those with mild, probably type II diabetes became pregnant at that time, and yet the maternal mortality was of the order of 30% and the perinatal mortality was 70% to 80%. With the introduction of insulin, young diabetic women lived long enough and were well enough to conceive, and the outlook improved. Nevertheless, as recently as 1949, Peel and Oakley (7) recorded a maternal mortality of 2.2% and a perinatal mortality of 40% in 458 cases treated in 25 teaching hospitals throughout the United Kingdom during the years 1942 through 1948. During the same period, they had treated 141 cases in their own clinic, with a 1.4% maternal loss and a 26% rate of perinatal loss. Since then, maternal mortality has been eliminated, and there has been a steady reduction in perinatal loss, as shown in the author's personal experience (Tables 9.3 and 9.4).

When these observations began in 1951, the advice of experts such as Peel and Oakley (7) was clear:

The risk of intrauterine death of the fetus rises gradually from the 32nd to the 40th week—after 36 weeks the risk of IUD exceeds that of NND (neonatal death). Therefore, in our view, 36 weeks is the optimum date for delivery.

This policy of premature delivery in the interest of the fetus was also applied by Priscilla White in Boston and by Jorgen Pedersen in Copenhagen. As far back as 1905, Jellett (8) of the Rotunda Hospital in Dublin had referred to premature delivery, but with a significant caveat:

It may sometimes be necessary to induce premature labour either for the sake of the mother or the child, but the indications are not plain and the *result is not promising*. [Emphasis added.]

TABLE 9.3. Personal series, Drury/ Dublin 1951–1985, Feb.

Viable infants	951	
Intrauterine deaths	38 }	71
Neonatal deaths ($\frac{1}{52}$)	33 }	
Perinatal loss rate 7.5%		

TABLE 9.4. Pregnancy in the pregestationally diabetic woman in Dublin.

Phase	No. of viables	No. of perinatal losses
1951–1974	502	49 (9.7%)
1975–1978*	154	8 (5.2%)
1979–1985(Feb.)[†]	295	14 (4.7%)
		(Excluding malformations = 3.1)

*Strict control + lecithin/sphingomyelin ratio.
[†]Strict control + late delivery.

How right he was that the results were not promising. In many cases this policy of premature delivery transferred the death from the stillborn to the neonatal category, since many of the infants died from hyaline membrane disease owing to lack of pulmonary surfactant. Nevertheless, the policy of premature delivery was continued and, indeed, is still practiced in many centers, albeit at a later stage of pregnancy.

Problems of Pregnancy in Women With Clinical Pregestational Diabetes

The problems peculiar to pregnancy in diabetic women may be considered under various headings:

Maternal

HYPOGLYCEMIA

Episodes of hypoglycemia are common in the first half of pregnancy and especially in the first trimester. This is due to the already mentioned combination of physiologic adaptations, the pursuit of strict control, and the nausea of early pregnancy. Patients and spouses (and neighbors) should be warned about this problem and instructed in the use of glucagon. Happily, the fetus tolerates hypoglycemia well. Indeed, I have records of 110 patients who experienced at least one episode of hypoglycemic coma without any related mishap to the fetus.

DIABETIC KETOACIDOSIS (DKA)

Since pregnancy has some features of the starvation state (see above), ketoacidosis is a real hazard. In contrast with hypoglycemia, it may be lethal to the fetus. In our own series there were 14 cases of DKA with 11 fetal deaths.

RETINOPATHY

Retinopathy is common at the onset of pregnancy and may progress as pregnancy advances. The progression of retinopathy may be related to strict metabolic control. In a prospective study of 53 patients, 33 (62%) had retinopathy when first examined and eight others (15%) developed it as pregnancy advanced. Progressive changes occurred as pregnancy advanced: microaneurysms increased moderately, hemorrhages appeared in 30 (56.6%), and soft exudation in 15 (28.3%). Four (7.5%) had neovascularization; one for the first time. Six months after delivery the background changes had regressed to control levels and neovascularization had regressed somewhat (9). As might be expected, the presence and progression of retinopathy were related to age at onset and to duration of diabetes. Thus, all patients who had diabetes for more than 10 years had some retinopathy. Neovascularization may be controlled by photocoagulation; in any case, retinopathy is not an indication for termination of pregnancy.

NEPHROPATHY

Nephropathy in the diabetic woman is defined as a persistent urinary excretion of more than 400 mg of protein per 24 hours during the first half of pregnancy, in the absence of urinary tract infection. Many patients will also have hypertension, elevated serum creatinine levels, and proliferative retinopathy; superimposed preeclamptic toxemia is common. Such cases demand meticulous supervision and control of both hypertension and diabetes, with early admission of the patient and premature delivery of the infant. In expert hands, the perinatal survival is 80%. Patients with functioning renal transplants have had successful pregnancies.

Fetal Problems

INTRAUTERINE DEATH

The spectre of unexpected (and often unexplained) intrauterine death has dominated the stage for many years and has determined the policy of premature delivery, which still influences much of the thinking behind management programs.

Hyperglycemia, erythremia, and cardiac malfunction in the fetus have all been considered possible causes of death. Although much less frequent today, such deaths still occur, as indeed they do also in nondiabetic pregnancies. They represent the main basis for the obsessional use of fetal-monitoring procedures.

MALFORMATIONS

Congenital anomalies occur in 6% to 8% of infants of diabetic mothers, that is, three times more frequently than in the general population. With the steady decline in perinatal mortality, the significance of deaths from malformations has increased and they now constitute about one in three of all perinatal deaths. The type of malformation covers a wide spectrum, but neural tube defects and heart lesions are especially common.

Kucera (10) compared the type and frequency of malformations in 340 infants born to diabetic mothers (4.8% were malformed) with a WHO survey of malformations in 7,104 infants born to nondiabetic mothers (1.65% were malformed). Mills et al (11) used the material to determine a ratio of incidences (relative frequency of the individual malformations within the collection of malformations) and, by using a developmental morphologic approach, to determine the time at which the defect occurred (Table 9.5). These authors concluded that "the insult causing malformations in IDM [infants of diabetic mothers] occurs before the seventh week" and that this insult "presumably relates to some aspect of the maternal milieu that is disturbed in diabetes." Further evidence that poor metabolic control in early pregnancy is associated with malformations is provided by Deuchar's work with rats (12) and by studies showing a correlation between high levels of maternal glycosylated hemoglobin in early pregnancy and congenital abnormalities. The obvious conclusion from these studies is that in women who report to the health care team after missing a period, the damage may already have been done. Therefore, diabetic women should be educated to report to their physician or clinic *when pregnancy is planned* so that the best possible control can be obtained before conception occurs. This approach *may* reduce the number of malformations, while ultrasonography and estimation of serum α-fetoprotein levels may detect the existence of neural tube defects.

TABLE 9.5. Congenital malformations in infants of women with diabetes mellitus.[10]

Anomaly	Ratio of incidences	Gestational age after ovulation in weeks
Caudal regression	252	3
Spina bifida: Hydrocephalus, etc.	2	4
Anencephalus	3	4
Heart anomalies	4	
Transposition of great vessels		5
Ventricular septal defect		6
Atrial septic defect		6
Anal-rectal atresia	3	6
Renal anomalies	5	
Agenesis	6	5
Cystic kidney	4	5
Ureter duplex	23	5
Situs inversus	84	4

Macrosomia

The original and simplistic view that macrosomia was due to maternal hyperglycemia causing β-cell hyperplasia in the fetus is incomplete; we have seen many macrosomic infants despite meticulous control of blood glucose levels. There may be a subset of euglycemic patients in whom levels of intermediate metabolites and amino acids are high enough to cause fetal β-cell hyperplasia. Macrosomic infants may cause difficulties at delivery, such as shoulder dystocia, and may experience considerable postnatal morbidity, such as hypoglycemia.

Small-for-Age Infants

Although the common perception is that neonates of patients with diabetes are macrosomic, some of them may be small for gestational age owing to intrauterine growth retardation, which is common in women with long-standing diabetes who have vascular complications. In this group the risk of intrauterine death has to be balanced against the risk associated with premature delivery.

Neonatal Morbidity

Respiratory Distress Syndrome

When patients were routinely delivered at 36 or 37 weeks gestation, inadequate amounts of pulmonary surfactant frequently resulted in a respiratory distress syndrome (RDS), which was often fatal. The measurement of the lecithin/sphingomyelin (L/S) ratio in the amniotic fluid, permitting the prediction of lung maturity, virtually eliminated this problem; other procedures, such as the foam stability test and the assays for desaturated phosphatidylcholine, phosphatidylglycerol, or lung surfactant apoproteins, may be more sensitive indicators (14).

Although the ability to predict pulmonary maturity is helpful, in our view its application has lost some of its relevance because uncomplicated, well-controlled patients should be delivered at term, making the test unnecessary. It is still of value when one is attempting to balance the risks of premature delivery versus delay in uncomplicated cases. Some cases of RDS appear to be due to diminished pulmonary compliance rather than to surfactant deficiency. Transient tachypnea of the newborn may arise from pulmonary edema, especially after cesarean section. Fortunately, respiratory problems not only are becoming much less frequent, but are more easily treated because of improvements in ventilation therapy.

Hypoglycemia

Neonatal hypoglycemia, defined as a blood glucose of less than 1.6 mmol/L (28.8 mg/dL) is common, especially in macrosomic infants. This association suggests a causative role for maternal hyperglycemia leading to β-cell hyperplasia in the fetus. After delivery, the hyperinsulinism persists and as the available glucose decreases, hypoglycemia occurs. This may be accentuated by a sluggish response of the counterregulatory system, i.e., deficient output of glucagon and catecholamines. Strict metabolic control in the mother and delayed delivery of the infant diminish the frequency and severity of neonatal hypoglycemia.

HYPERBILIRUBINEMIA

Defined as a level of plasma bilirubin in excess of 15 mg/dL, hyperbilirubinemia is clearly related to premature delivery and inadequate maturation of liver enzymes, which conjugate bilirubin. If there is significant erythremia, the degree of bilirubinemia will be greater still. Treatment is by phototherapy. Erythremia, hyperviscosity, hypocalcemia, and hypomagnesemia may also occur in the infant of the diabetic mother. There is no clear explanation for these abnormalities, but they are seen more often in infants delivered prematurely.

Summary

Some of the aforementioned problems are inherent to diabetes, such as maternal hypoglycemia in early pregnancy, increased tendency for maternal ketoacidosis, increased frequency of polyhydramnios and toxemia, inexplicable intrauterine death, and marked increase in congenital malformations. Strict maternal metabolic control will markedly diminish all of these, with the exception of maternal hypoglycemia, which it may, in fact, increase. Other problems stem from the policies that are advocated in an effort to eliminate intrauterine deaths, such as early admission, intensive monitoring, premature delivery, and frequent use of cesarean section.

Fetal Surveillance, Timing of Delivery, and Third Trimester Management—According to the Experts

The indiscriminate use of fetal surveillance procedures inevitably results in premature deliveries and high rates of cesarean section-induced perinatal morbidity. The economic and social costs are considerable. Yet, many have written dogmatically in support of these regimes. For example:

Intensive, expensive programs of fetal monitoring must be used to prevent stillbirths (15).

The objective at the author's center is to permit pregnancy in the diabetic woman to be carried near to term (38–40 weeks) unless fetal health becomes compromised. We are currently evaluating the need for early admission in the light of present advances in the monitoring of mother and fetus. While this assessment is underway, we continue to admit patients early and to allow pregnancies to proceed to term unless complications arise. [and, further] Diabetic women in White Class D, F and R are admitted to hospital at 32 weeks, those in White Class C at 34 weeks and White Class B at 36 weeks. Daily collections of urine are made for estriol levels; non-stress contraction tests are performed only when non-stress tests are abnormal; amniocenteses are performed at 32 weeks and repeated at 38 weeks if immature patterns are found (16).

Our insulin-dependent patients are admitted to the hospital at 36 weeks gestation for intensive fetal monitoring and control of diabetes. . . . In the hospital, daily estriol measurements are made and the non-stress test is performed twice weekly. . . . It is impossible to determine which aspect of our program is responsible for success, i.e., better diabetic control or use of fetal monitoring tests. However, such a program certainly has allowed pregnancies to be carried to term without fetal jeopardy. In the future, it may be possible for very well-controlled diabetic women to remain outside the hospital until 38 weeks gestation but *this idea has not been tested* (17). [Emphasis added.]

Once labor is underway *it is imperative* [emphasis added] that continuous fetal heart rate monitoring with scalp pH back-up be performed since the incidence of intrapartum fetal distress (persistent late decelerations and scalp pH <7.25) is high in diabetic pregnancy (18).

Such unanimity among the experts might suggest that they must be right and that to disagree would be foolhardy. Nevertheless, it is always important for the questioning voice to be heard. It seems to me that the "thinking" behind management programs is still dominated by the traditional view that the fetus in the womb of every diabetic mother is at risk and that every available means must be used to monitor its well-being and the integrity of the placenta. If the information thus obtained dominates rather than serves to complement clinical judgment, a high rate of intervention will result. Paradoxically, the availability of the L/S ratio, etc encourages this.

Although my description of the scenario may be argued, the facts are beyond dispute: in 11 reports dealing with 1,116 diabetic mothers published in the United States between 1977 and 1983 with a perinatal loss of 5.2%, the cesarean section rate varied from 54% to 80%, and an article in a journal published by the American Diabetes Association declares that:

Currently, intensive antepartum surveillance methods are used, in a variety of regimens, to identify the fetus in jeopardy and in need of delivery as well as those whose delivery can be postponed until maturity. These methods include daily estriol measurements (urine or plasma), weekly or biweekly stress tests . . ., serial sonography. . . . Most perinatologists agree that these tests should be used in combination because of unacceptable false positive rates from any test used alone. The time to initiate these tests, the frequency of testing, the location of testing (outpatient or hospital) and the specific tests used, if any, vary from center to center. However, all agree that in the well-controlled woman with a normally grown fetus it is safe to delay delivery until fetal maturity occurs (if all tests remain negative) (19).

In light of these recommendations one might reasonably expect that a substantial number of patients would be delivered at term and, as a corollary, that the cesarean section rate would not be high. However, such expectations are not realized, for the authors then tell us that:

Approximately 80% of women at our hospital are delivered by CS, the route of delivery in 60% to 90% of women with diabetes antedating pregnancy in US today. CS allows safe delivery of large infants and early delivery among women whose cervices are unfavorable for induction (20).

What conclusions can one draw from this apparent contradiction? It seems unlikely that so many patients would be in jeopardy. In fact, we know from our own experience that this is not so. Is it possible, therefore, that "intensive antepartum surveillance measures" are so unreliable or beget such anxiety among the obstetricians that instead of selecting the small number of patients in whom preterm delivery is indicated, they create a situation in which the intervention rate becomes alarmingly high? An alternative explanation is that there is a conscious or unconscious commitment to early intervention and planned cesarian section.

Is there an alternative approach? We suggest that in well-controlled, uncomplicated patients, good clinical supervision is adequate and that intensive surveillance be reserved for cases in which there are clinical grounds for anxiety. This conservative approach is practiced in the Dublin Maternity Hospitals in which I work, with the results outlined in Tables 9.3 and 9.4, and is based on a management program that started in 1951, evolved with time, and is described in the following section.

Timing of Delivery and Third-Trimester Management—According to Drury

First Visit

At first visit (preferably before conception), the importance of regular attendance and strict metabolic control is emphasized. We aim to maintain the blood glucose levels at 5 to 7 mmol/L (90 to 126 mg/dL), using twice-daily injections of a mixture of fast- and intermediate-acting insulins. Each patient estimates and records the capillary blood glucose four to six times daily and is taught to make appropriate adjustments in insulin dosage. At fortnightly (first 20 weeks) or weekly (second 20 weeks, or if control is inadequate) visits, the patient brings three or four venous samples (collected by patient, spouse, or district nurse) for blood glucose estimations in our laboratory. These samples are collected at the following times: fasting, midmorning, midafternoon, and bedtime. At each clinic visit the glycosylated hemoglobin is also estimated. Ideally, this program should be initiated before conception.

Team Effort

The clinic is a joint one at which a physician and an obstetrician see the patient together. The obstetrician records regularly his impression of fetal size and may use ultrasonography to assess gestational age and fetal size. Antenatal cardiotocography and tests of placental function are reserved for patients who develop obstetrical complications or whose metabolic control is unsatisfactory. We do not admit patients routinely at any stage of pregnancy (21). Thus, in a series of 141 consecutive pregnancies managed in the National Maternity Hospital, only one third of the patients spent a short time in the hospital because of inadequate control. All who developed polyhydramnios or hypertension with proteinuria were admitted. Ultrasonography was performed in the first trimester in 34 patients to assist in the determination of gestational age. Twice-weekly serial urinary estrogen determinations (52 in all) were performed in 12 patients who either had hypertension with proteinuria or in whom fetal growth retardation was suspected.

Ticket to Go to Term

Uncomplicated cases in good metabolic control are allowed to go to term. If spontaneous labor does not occur at that time, the membranes are ruptured. Twenty hours later an oxytocin infusion is initiated if labor has not begun. Six hours later the patient is delivered by cesarean section if by then delivery is not imminent; the policy being to achieve delivery within 30 hours of rupture of the membranes. In the series mentioned above, electronic fetal monitoring was used only in five cases where clear amniotic fluid was not demonstrated. The L/S ratio is measured only in cases in which premature delivery is contemplated.

Results of Conservative Management

Reference to Table 9.4 shows that in 295 consecutive pregnancies managed between 1979 and 1984, there were 14 perinatal deaths (4.7%). Excluding five malformations (Table 9.6), the perinatal loss was nine in 290 pregnancies, i.e., 3.1%.

TABLE 9.6. 295 viable infants: perinatal loss 14 (4.7%) (Personal series, Drury/Dublin 1979–985, Feb.).

1 iniencephaly, 3 anencephaly, 1 multiple.

Excluding 5 malformations.

Corrected perinatal loss $\dfrac{9}{290} = 3.1\%$

TABLE 9.7. Perinatal deaths, excluding 8 malformations = 11 (3.1%) (Dublin 1979–1986, May 358 cases).

White's class	A1	at Wk.	Details
C	—	—	Referred at 25 wks. Bad control. IUD at 35 wks. 526 g.
B	9.4	10	Admitted in labor. 36 wks. F.H.N.H. Anoxia 1,680 g.
D	8	7	Deaf, polychondritis, active hepatitis, steroids. Rhesus due to transfusion. L.S. 1.6. IUD at 36 wks. Autopsy indicated that death was due to rhesus problem.
B	14.7	10	Intermittent proteinuria 139–90. Excess liquor. Heavy smoker. IUD at 37 weeks and 5 days.
D	9.8	23	Hydramnios. A.R.M. at 39 wks. Obstructed labor. Failed forceps. CS too late. 5,130 g.
F/R	13.3	10	Essential hypertension. Growth retard. IUD at 32 wks. 850 g.
D	10.4	14	160/100 blood pressure. Proteinuria 2 g. in 24 h. Cigarettes 40. C.T.G. misread. IUD at 35 wks. 3,230 g.
D	12.3	10	IUD 32 wks. 1,984 g.
B	8.9	5	IUD 35 wks. 2,760 g.
C	15.1	36(?)	DM for 5 years. Stopped insulin a year before. Reported at ? 36 wks. FBG = 16.6 Fructosamine = 3.19 (normal < 1.4) IUD soon after initiation of treatment.
B	9.9	15	Unsuitable for induction at 39 wks. IUD at 39½ wks. Macerated and macrosomic.

IUD, intrauterine deaths; FHNH, fetal heart not heard; ARM, artificial rupture of membrane; CTG, cardiotocograph; FBG, fasting blood glucose I, 16.6 mmol/L.

Perinatal morbidity was low (Table 9.8) because of the policy of late delivery (Table 9.9). For the same reason there was a high rate of spontaneous labor and of successful induction with a corresponding high rate of vaginal delivery (74%) and a low rate of cesarean section (26%) (Table 9.10). Even in primigravidae, the cesarean section rate was only 32%. The low rate of perinatal morbidity allows us to send many babies directly to the postnatal ward with the mother, a policy that facilitates maternal-infant bonding.

TABLE 9.8. Neonatal morbidity in live born infants.

Condition	%
Jaundice	13.6
Hypoglycemia	10.4
Transient tachypnea	8.0
Infection	4.8
Respiratory distress syndrome	2.4
Meconium aspiration	1.6
Seizures	1.6

TABLE 9.9. Time of delivery in 284 patients (i.e. 295 less 11 intrauterine deaths) in which no decision about time of delivery was irrelevant. (Dublin 1979–1985, Feb.).

Time	Number	%
Before 38 wks	52	(18.3)
38–38 %⁷	75	(26.4)
39–39 %⁷	60	(21.1)
40–	97	(34.2)

IUD, intrauterine death.

TABLE 9.10. Dublin 1979–1985, Feb., 284 deliveries.

Vaginal delivery	74%
*Cesarean section	26%

*One half were primary elective.

Perinatal Mortality

During the period 1979 to May 1986 there were 19 perinatal deaths in 358 pregnancies. Eight of these were due to malformations, which continue to constitute the hard core of perinatal loss. It is possible that a greater effort toward preconceptual metabolic control may reduce this loss. The remaining 11 perinatal deaths are detailed in Table 9.7.

Conclusions

Although a number of these deaths might have been avoided by earlier delivery or by cesarean section, this does not invalidate the notion that in uncomplicated well-controlled cases, clinical surveillance with ultrasonography is adequate and that spontaneous labor at term may be awaited. We believe, therefore, that it is possible to avoid prolonged expensive hospitalization, which also disrupts family life, and that "intensive, expensive programs of fetal monitoring" are in most cases unnecessary.

References

1. Steinke J, Driscoll SG (1965) The extractable insulin content of pancreas from foetuses and infants of diabetic and control mothers. Diabetes. 14:573–578.
2. Freinkel N (1964) Effect of the conceptus on maternal metabolism during pregnancy—On the nature of treatment of diabetes Leibel BS, Wrenshall GA (eds): Excerpta Medica, Amsterdam, 679–700.
3. WHO Expert Committee on Diabetes Mellitus (1980)—second report. Tech. Rep. Serv. WHO, p 646.
4. National Diabetes Data Group (1979) Classification and diagnosis of DM and other categories of glucose intolerance. Diabetes 28:1039–1057.
5. O'Sullivan JB, Mahan CM (1964) Criteria for the OGTT in pregnancy. Diabetes 13:278–285.
6. Jarrett RJ (1951) Reflections on Gestational Diabetes Mellitus. Lancet 2:1220–1222.
7. Peel JH, Oakley WG (1949) The 12th Br. Cong. of Obst. and Gynecol.
8. Jellett IJ (1905) Manual of Midwifery. Bailliere Tindall & Cox, London, p 580.

9. Drury MI, Moloney JBM (1982) The effect of pregnancy on the natural history of Diabetes Retinopathy. Am J Opthalmol 93:745–756.
10. Kucera J (1971) Rate and Type of congenital anomalies among offspring of diabetic women. J Reprod Med 7:61–70.
11. Mills JL, Baker L, Goldman AS (1979) Malformations in infants of diabetic mothers occur before the 7th gestational week. Diabetes 28:292–293.
12. Deuchar E (1978) Carbohydrate metabolism in pregnancy and the newborn, in Sutherland HW, Stovers JW (eds): Second Aberdeen Collaquium. Berlin, Springer-Verlag, pp 247–263.
13. Miller E, Hare JW, Cloherty JP, et al (1981) Elevated HbA1 in early pregnancy and major congenital anomalies in IDM. N Engl Med 304:1331–1334.
14. Katyal SL, Amenta JS, Singh G, Silverman JA (1981) Deficient lung surfactant apoproteins in amniotic fluid with mature phospholipid profile from diabetic pregnancies. Am J Obstet Gynecol 148-1:48–53.
15. Kitzmiller JL, Cloherty JP, Graham CA (1982) Clinical Diabetes Mellitus. WB Saunders, Philadelphia, p 203.
16. Freinkel N, Metzer BE, Potter JM (1983) Diabetes Mellitus. Medical Examination Publishing Co Inc, New York. p 704.
17. Kitzmiller JL, Cloherty JP, Graham CA (1982) Clinical Diabetes Mellitus. WB Saunders, Philadelphia p 210.
18. Kitzmiller JL, Cloherty JP, Graham CA (1982) Clinical Diabetes Mellitus. WB Saunders, Philadelphia. p 212.
19. Whalley PJ, Leveno KJ (1984) The Diabetic Pregnancy: Issues in Management, Essentials of Care. Am J Obstet Gynecol 2-3:51–55.
20. Whalley PJ, Leveno KJ (1984) The Diabetic Pregnancy: Issues in Management, Essentials of Care. Am J Obstet Gynecol 2-4:82–83.
21. Drury MI, Stronge JM, Foley ME, et al (1983) Pregnancy in the Diabetic Patient: Timing and Mode of Delivery. Obstet Gynaec 62, 3:279–282.

Part V   Infant Outcome of Pregnancies Complicated by Diabetes

10
The Metabolic Sequelae in the Infant of the Diabetic Mother

RICHARD M. COWETT

Introduction

From a developmental standpoint, the normal newborn is in a transitional state relative to glucose homeostasis. The delivery of glucose to the fetus depends on the mother, whose glucose homeostasis as an adult is regulated to a fine degree (1). In contrast, maintenance of glucose homeostasis may be a major problem even in the normal newborn (2). This is because the newborn must provide for energy (particularly for the brain, which consumes 70% of glucose production per kilogram per minute) and growth while maintaining a balance between continuous glucose needs and intermittent oral intake. Thus, homeostasis depends on a balance between substrate availability and developing hormone (insulin and contra-insulin hormones), neural, and enzymatic systems. The precarious nature of this balance is emphasized by the frequent occurrence of neonatal hypoglycemia or hyperglycemia and associated morbidities, especially in the infant of the diabetic mother (IDM). Although study of the IDM has provided much information about the pathophysiology of glucose homeostasis, the discussion that follows shows how much additional work needs to be done. The problem has been discussed in a number of extensive reviews (3,4).

Although many IDMs have an uneventful perinatal course, there is still an increased risk of complications, which can be minimized with appropriate obstetric and pediatric care. This chapter evaluates many of the difficulties that an IDM may encounter, analyzes the pathophysiologic basis for their occurrence, and outlines specific rationale for treatment.

Perinatal Mortality and Morbidity

Infants of diabetic mothers have greater morbidity than infants of non-diabetic mothers. Many infants of women with insulin-dependent diabetes, and an even greater number of infants of women with gestational diabetes experience an uneventful clinical course (5). Theoretically, the more rigorous the metabolic control of the mother is, the greater is the potential for a normal infant. Indeed, except for congenital anomalies, the perinatal mortality of IDM approaches that of infants of nondiabetic mothers (6,7).

The physician responsible for the care and delivery of the mother must inform the physician responsible for the care of the infant well in advance of delivery, because knowledge of the character of the maternal diabetes, prior pregnancy history, and complications occurring during pregnancy will allow the physician caring for the infant to anticipate many of the potential fetal and neonatal complications (Table 10.1) and to be present at delivery.

Studies of perinatal morbidity and mortality from diverse centers attest to the increasing success of the above principles. In 1974 Pedersen et al published an analysis of their 26-year experiences with 1,332 diabetic pregnancies (8). Perinatal mortality varied directly with the severity of maternal diabetes as judged by White's original classification of diabetes in pregnancy and by Pedersen's "prognostically bad signs in pregnancy" (PBSP) classification. White's subsequently revised classification is based on the duration of diabetes (Table 10.2) and on the presence of vascular complications (9), while the PBSP classification (Table 10.3) includes abnormalities occuring during the current pregnancy. The risk to the fetus was increased when the two classifications were combined. These investigators noted that although the neonatal outcome in diabetic pregnancy had also improved during the same period, the improved classification combined with increased experience was the major reason for the improved outcome in the diabetic pregnancy. This improved perinatal mortality has been confirmed at many centers in the United States and in Europe, but

TABLE 10.1. Potential morbidity in the infant of the diabetic mother.

Asphyxia
Birth injury
Congenital anomalies
Heart failure
Hyperbilirubinemia
Hypocalcemia
Hypoglycemia
Hypomagnesemia
Increased blood volume
Macrosomia
Neurologic instability
Organomegaly
Erythremia and hyperviscosity
Respiratory distress and respiratory distress syndrome
Small left colon syndrome
Transient hematuria

TABLE 10.2. White's classification of diabetes in pregnancy (modified).

Gestational diabetes	Abnormal glucose tolerance test; euglycemia maintained by diet alone or with insulin required
Class A	Diet alone, any duration or age of onset
Class B	Onset age 20 years or older and duration less than 10 years
Class C	Onset age 10 to 19 years or duration 10 to 19 years
Class D	Onset age under 10 years, duration over 20 years, background retinopathy, or hypertension (not preeclampsia)
Class R	Proliferative retinopathy
Class F	Nephropathy with proteinuria over 500 mg a day
Class RF	Criteria for R and F coexist
Class H	Arteriosclerotic heart disease clinically evident
Class T	Prior renal transplantation

From Hare JW, White P, reference 9. Reproduced with permission from the American Diabetes Association, Inc.

although the frequency of macrosomia also has decreased, the rate is still higher than that in infants born to nondiabetic women. A recent survey showed that most macrosomic infants were born to obese mothers, not all of whom had glucose intolerance, as judged by postpartum glyco-hemoglobin determinations (10,11). Nevertheless, gestational diabetes developing late in pregnancy often remains undiagnosed, thus increasing the risk of perinatal complications.

A recent evaluation of perinatal mortality has been published by Teramo et al (12). Their study covered two time periods separated by a change in the systems of maternal and neonatal care, involving increased monitoring and more frequent hospitalization for metabolic control, especially in the third trimester. During the second period (1975 through 1977) all diabetic patients were hospitalized from the 32 nd week of pregnancy until delivery. Strict maintenance of normoglycemia (blood glucose <120 mg/dL) was the goal of management, and in the latter years, a permanent interdisciplinary team was in charge of the patient. The results were a significant increase in the gestational age of the infants without an increase in mean birth weight and a marked fall in perinatal mortality and neonatal morbidity. The authors concluded that although progress was obvious, a significant neonatal morbidity was still present.

Similar conclusions about the value of strict metabolic control were reached by Jerwell et al who evaluated their experience with 1,035 births to diabetic mothers between 1957 and 1976 (13). During this 10-year period, not only did the perinatal mortality fall by 30%, but the duration of ges-

TABLE 10.3. Poor prognostic signs in pregnancy.

Pyelonephritis
Precoma or severe acidosis
Toxemia
"Neglectors"

From Pedersen J, reference 17.

tation increased from 35.5 to 37 weeks and the number of infants whose weight was appropriate for gestational age increased from 53.3% to 70.0%. These results were attributed to improved care of the diabetic woman resulting from increased referral to university clinics and regional hospitals (from 38.7% in 1967 through 1968 to 77.1% in 1975 through 1976). Improved care did not affect the rate of malformations, which was still 50% more common among infants born to diabetic women than in the general population.

A recent study of 154 pregnant diabetic patients, hospitalized for a month prior to delivery, showed that although there was a significant association between maternal glucose variability and neonatal outcome (but not between maternal glucose variability and the birth weight of the infant), absence of variability did not insure against neonatal complications (14).

Another attempt to maintain normoglycemia in diabetic women with vascular complications resulted in some improvement of proteinuria and retinopathy; however, neonatal macrosomia was still observed despite normal maternal hemoglobin A_{1c} levels (15).

Coustan and Imarah obtained a partial decline in the incidence of macrosomia, operative delivery, and birth trauma by means of more rigorous metabolic control in women with gestational diabetes (16).

Thus, maintenance of euglycemia appears to diminish, but not completely eradicate, the increased perinatal and neonatal mortality and morbidity noted in the diabetic pregnancy. The possible reasons for this are discussed below.

Effects of Maternal Diabetes on the Fetus

As yet, no single pathogenetic mechanism for the diverse problems observed in IDMs has been clearly identified. Nevertheless, many of the effects can be attributed to defective maternal metabolic (glucose) control. Pedersen originally emphasized the relationship between maternal glucose concentration and neonatal hypoglycemia (Table 10.4) and suggested that fetal hyperglycemia secondary to maternal hyperglycemia stimulated the fetal pancreas, resulting in islet cell hypertrophy, β-cell hyperplasia, and increased insulin production (17). Upon separation of the fetus from the

TABLE 10.4. Evidence of "hyperinsulinism" in IDM.

Islet hyperplasia and β-cell hypertrophy
Obesity and macrosomia
Hypoglycemia with low free fatty acids
Rapid glucose disappearance rate
   Increased plasma insulin response to glucose
    High levels of immunoreactive insulin in the umbililcal blood
Increased levels of plasma C-peptide and proinsulin

mother, the former, no longer supported by placental glucose transfer, may develop hypoglycemia. In addition, since insulin is the primary anabolic hormone of fetal growth and development, hyperinsulinism in utero results in visceromegaly (especially heart and liver), increased muscle mass, and, in the presence of excess substrate (glucose), increased fat synthesis and deposition, especially during the third trimester (18,19). After delivery there is a rapid fall in plasma glucose, with persistently low concentrations of plasma free fatty acids, glycerol, and β-hydroxybutyrate. The response of plasma immunoreactive insulin and C-peptide to an intravenous glucose stimulus is increased (20), and so is the insulin response to intravenous arginine (21). On the other hand, while the initial response to an oral glucose load is more prompt, the total response, as determined by the area under the insulin curve, is not increased (22). During the initial hours after birth, the rate of glucose disappearance from the plasma after an intravenous bolus is faster in IDM than in normal infants (23). In contrast, following stepwise hourly increments in the rate of glucose infusion, the plasma glucose concentration increases following infusion at the normal rate of 4 to 6 mg/kg/min (24,25), possibly secondary to the persistence of hepatic glucose output similar to that of the normal infant.

Plasma glucocorticoids and growth hormone levels do not appear to change significantly in IDMs. Studies of the somatomedins (IGF$_1$, IGF$_2$) are being evaluated presently. In contrast, urinary excretion of catecholamines is diminished, especially in infants with low plasma glucose concentration (26), and the neonatal rise in plasma glucagon is less pronounced than in normal infants (27).

A recent study suggests that monocytes isolated from the placental blood of infants of gestationally diabetic mothers at delivery have more insulin receptors than do the monocytes of normal adults or normal infants and that the number and affinity of these receptors increase rather than decrease with increasing concentrations of plasma insulin (28). The physiologic significance of these observations is unclear, although they may portend a further enhancement of insulin action.

Kinetic Analysis of Glucose Metabolism in IDM

In vivo kinetic analysis has been used by numerous investigators for the metabolic evaluation of IDMs. Thus, Kalhan et al used infusions of glucose labeled with ^{13}C, a stable nonradioactive isotope, to measure systemic glucose production rates in five normal infants of nondiabetic women and in five infants of insulin-dependent diabetic women at two hours of age (29). As expected, the IDMs had lower glucose concentrations than the infants of the normal mothers, but, in addition, the IDMs had lower rates of glucose production. The authors speculated that this decrease was due to an inhibition of glycogenolysis, possibly related to an increased insulin and a decreased glucagon and catecholamine response. What is fascinating about this report is that these diabetic women, having been hospitalized during the last 4 weeks of pregnancy, had achieved what was considered excellent metabolic control according to the standards of the time (blood glucose between 50 and 150 mg/dL). Nevertheless, the glucose production rates in their infants were lower than that in control infants.

Five years later (1982) the same group of investigators (30) again measured glucose production in five infants of "strictly controlled" insulin-dependent diabetic mothers, in one infant of a gestational diabetic woman, and in five infants born to normal mothers. The maternal blood glucose levels were in a range (36 to 164 mg/dL) similar to that of the previous series, and the mothers were hospitalized for 3 to 4 weeks before delivery. In this series, the basal rate of glucose production was similar in the infants of diabetic and nondiabetic women. However, in the infants of the diabetic women it was not as effectively suppressed by an infusion of glucose as

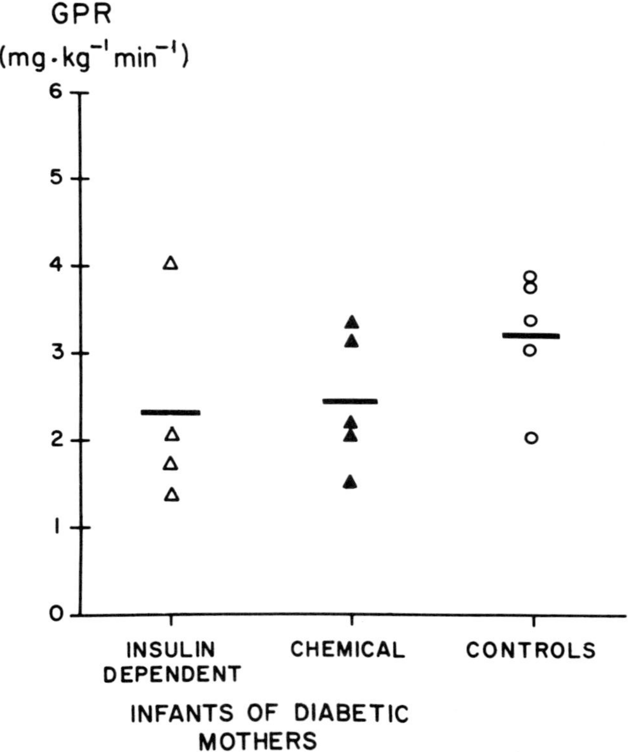

FIGURE 10.1. Glucose production rates in the three groups of infants studied. (From Cowett et al (32) with permission.)

it was in the normal ones. These results are similar to those we have obtained in the infants of nine diabetic women (four insulin-dependent, five noninsulin dependent) and in five infants of normal women (31,32) (Figure 10.1), in which we found that the rate of glucose production in the neonate is variable (33). These data parallel other work from the same group which reflect the transitional nature of glucose metabolism in the term and preterm infant (33).

The notion that neonatal glucose homeostasis is in a transitional state is further supported by studies in which the metabolic control of gestationally diabetic women was evaluated in relation to the birth weights of the infants (34). Contrary to Pedersen's hypothesis, no correlation between birth weight and mean maternal plasma glucose concentration during the third trimester of pregnancy was found in this group of gestational diabetic women (Figure 10.2). Similar findings led Freinkel, Milner, and others to suggest that the normal mixture of nutrients (amino acids, free fatty acids, etc) rather than glucose alone is crucial in the regulation of fetal β-cell function (Figure 10.3) (35,36).

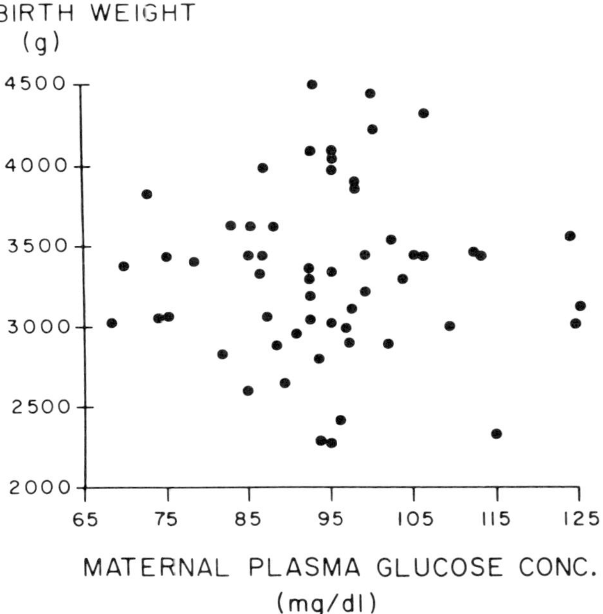

FIGURE 10.2. Correlation between birth weight and mean maternal plasma concentration (mg/dl) during the last trimester of pregnancy in the glucose-intolerant group. (From Widness et al (34). Reproduced with permission from the American Diabetes Association, Inc.)

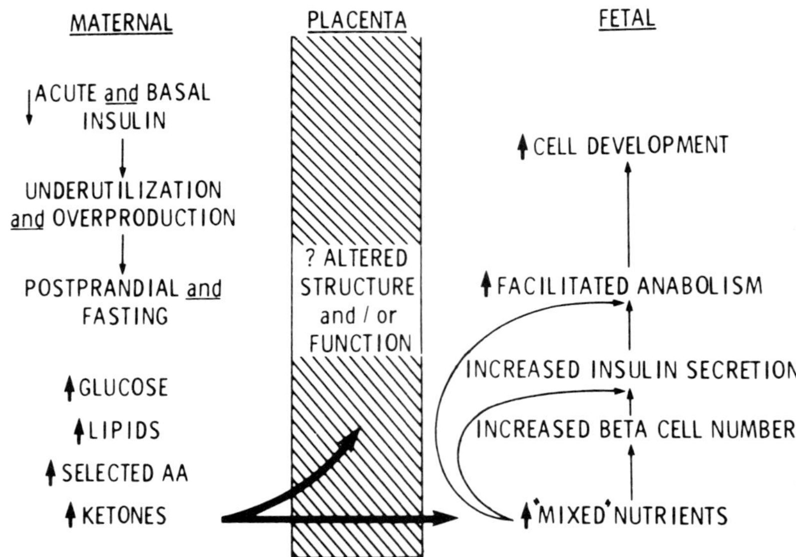

FIGURE 10.3. Fetal development in insulinogenic diabetic pregnancy utilizing maternal mixed nutrients as controlling factors. (From Freinkel (35). Reproduced with permission from the American Diabetes Association, Inc.)

Congenital Anomalies

Although definite progress is being made in the control of morbidity and mortality in the IDM, congenital abnormalities continue to occur three to four times more frequently in the offspring of diabetic women and remain the most frequent cause of perinatal mortality (7,12,37,38). This is true even in those centers where the perinatal mortality due to causes other than congenital malformations is not greater in the offspring of diabetic women than in the offspring of nondiabetic women (6,39).

The reason for the increased incidence of congenital anomalies in IDMs is obscure, although several hypotheses have been proposed. Among them are 1) maternal hyperglycemia, either before or after conception, 2) maternal hypoglycemia, 3) fetal hyperinsulinemia, 4) uteroplacental vascular disease, and/or 5) genetic predisposition. Although there are data to support all of the above, the most likely etiologic factor appears to be postconception hyperglycemia.

If genetic factors were operative, one might anticipate that offspring of diabetic fathers and nondiabetic mothers would have an increased incidence of congenital anomalies. However, a review of 1,262 offspring of diabetic fathers revealed only a slight increase in anomalies of questionable significance, in contrast to a marked increase in the offspring of diabetic mothers (40). Unfortunately, information about the relationship between maternal hyperglycemia and fetal anomalies is still scant, perhaps because organogenesis takes place at a time during pregnancy when many diabetic women are not carefully evaluated for hyperglycemia. The importance of strict control of maternal diabetes has been emphasized repeatedly. Thus, one group of workers reported that a therapeutic regimen started before the women knew that they were pregnant markedly reduced the incidence of congenital anomalies (41). Another report indicates that a group of insulin-dependent women with high Hb A_{1c} values during the first trimester of pregnancy were more likely to give birth to babies with congenital anomalies (42). The importance of early control of maternal blood glucose is emphasized by two other recent studies. One of them (43) demonstrated that a group of women with insulin-dependent juvenile-onset diabetes in whom insulin therapy had been carefully adjusted preconceptually had no malformed offspring, whereas the rate of malformation was 9.6% in a similar group of women who had not received the benefit of such intensified treatment. The second study (44) suggested that good control started after the first trimester did not decrease the incidence of congenital malformations, although other types of morbidity did decrease. In fact, the neonatal malformation rate rose and was not influenced by maternal age or type of diabetes.

Hypoglycemia, a frequent occurrence in pregnant women with insulin-dependent diabetes, may also play a teratogenic role. If so, the mechanism of teratogenesis is unclear, because even though the injection of insulin into chick embryos causes severe malformations (45), current data indicate that the primate placenta is an effective barrier to the transfer of maternal insulin (46,47).

The increase in anomalies with increasing duration and severity of diabetes (according to White's classification) suggests that maternal vascular disease may also play a role (17). Although anomalies in the offspring of diabetic mothers involve several organ systems and do not constitute a specific syndrome, certain patterns tend to occur more frequently. A rare congenital defect is the small left colon syndrome, a condition that usually resolves spontaneously within the neonatal period. Its etiology is obscure, although it occurs more frequently in IDMs (48). More common are major congenital heart disease; musculoskeletal deformities, including the caudal regression syndrome; and central nervous system deformities (anencephaly, spina bifida, hydrocephalus). These findings indicate that the critical period of teratogenesis occurs before the seventh week of gestation.

A recent report describes 11 IDMs who presented with signs of respiratory distress. All had echocardiographic evidence of septal hypertrophy (49). In this group of patients the symptoms disappeared within 2 to 4 weeks, and the hypertrophy resolved within 2 to 12 months. Another study describes 34 infants of diabetic mothers with hypertrophy of the interventricular septum and of the right and left ventricular walls (50). Hypertrophy was seen more frequently in infants whose mothers were under poor diabetic control. Similar conclusions were reached by a third group of workers who noted septal hypertrophy in six of 18 infants of diabetic mothers. These six had profound hypoglycemia after birth, in contrast to the 12 infants without hypertrophy, who did not (51). The findings are consistent with the notion that fetal hyperinsulinism contributes directly to septal hypertrophy. Chronic hyperinsulinemia induced in the fetus of the rhesus monkey appears to be associated with significant muscular hypertrophy and cardiomegaly (19).

Although cardiac hypertrophy has been noted in autopsies of IDMs for the past three decades, it has only been in the last 5 years that attention has been directed to a peculiar form of subaortic stenosis, sometimes associated with symptomatic congestive heart failure, similar to idiopathic hypertrophic subaortic stenosis of the adult (52). As in the adult, therapy with digoxin is contraindicated, as it causes a potentially deleterious increase in myocardial contractility. Propranolol appears to be the drug of choice. Clinically, this disorder, as well as its ECG features, resolves spontaneously over a period of weeks or months.

Finally, an epidemiologic study of 2,587 newborn infants of diabetic mothers carried out between 1926 and 1983 revealed an overall malformation rate of 6.6%. The series was divided into five consecutive periods representing 500 infants each. During the final period of study, between 1979 and 1983, the authors noted a decrease in severity and frequency of congenital malformations. Interestingly, they also reported that fetuses statistically smaller than normal in early pregnancy had a higher risk of being malformed and concluded that preconception metabolic control is necessary for optimal fetal outcome (53).

Macrosomia, Birth Injury, and Asphyxia

The newborn infant of the poorly controlled diabetic patient often will appear macrosomic, in contrast with the infant born to the well-controlled diabetic and the nondiabetic, nonobese mother. If undetected, macrosomia may complicate vaginal delivery and result in asphyxia and/or birth injuries, such as cephalhematoma, subdural hemorrhage, facial palsy, ocular hemorrhage, clavicular fracture, and brachial plexus injuries (3,4). In addition, damage to the phrenic nerve may result in diaphragmatic paralysis, while the associated organomegaly may cause hemorrhage in the abdominal organs and, in particular, in the liver and the adrenal glands. Hemorrhage into the external genitalia has also been reported. To minimize these risks, intrapartum monitoring and careful neonatal evaluation of asphyxia are essential. Apgar scores should be determined one and five minutes after birth. Asphyxia may cause delayed respiratory difficulties or acute malfunction of the respiratory, renal, and central nervous systems.

Thus, decreased fluid intake is usually recommended until the degree of injury to the renal and central nervous systems can be ascertained.

Current management of the pregnant diabetic woman includes determining the degree of pulmonary maturity by measuring the lecithin/sphingomyelin (L/S) ratio, the presence of phosphatidylglycerol, and/or foam stability test (FST). In interpreting the results of these tests, one must keep in mind that a false positive L/S ratio may be associated with asphyxia. Indeed, a study of 150 women who had amniocentesis within 72 hours of delivery and whose L/S ratio was 2:1 demonstrated that the incidence of respiratory distress syndrome was significantly higher in infants who had low Apgar scores one and five minutes after birth, regardless of whether the mother had diabetes mellitus or not (54).

A rare occurrence of neonatal gangrene of the upper extremity with massive muscle necrosis of the forearm in the infant of a diabetic mother was recently reported (55). Sixty similar cases had been reported previously. It was postulated that gangrene was the result of a propensity for thrombosis in the IDM.

It may be concluded that early identification of maternal diabetes and maintenance of good metabolic control should diminish the frequency and magnitude of macrosomia and its attendant complications, and careful obstetric management should prevent birth injury and asphyxia.

Respiratory Distress Syndrome

Respiratory distress, including the respiratory distress syndrome (RDS), is a frequent and potentially severe complication in the IDM. Although the clinical association has been long recognized, recent investigations have increased our understanding of the pathophysiologic interrelationships. Neonatal RDS (pathologic correlate: hyaline membrane disease) develops because of lung immaturity and remains a major cause of mortality in the newborn.

Respiratory distress syndrome has a typical course that is manifest by increasing oxygen requirements owing to progressive respiratory compromise. Tachypnea, intercostal and subcostal retractions, nasal flaring, and expiratory grunting appearing in the first few minutes or hours of life, are the cardinal signs of the disease. In uncomplicated cases the disease peaks by 72 hours of age. Complications commonly associated with the disease include persistent patent ductus arteriosus in the very small (<1,500 g) infant and bronchopulmonary dysplasia requiring prolonged ventilatory support and high ambient oxygen concentrations. Both complications may significantly lengthen the clinical course of an otherwise self-limited disease. Lack of surfactant produced by type II pneumocytes, which normally decrease surface tension at the air to alveolar interface, results in pulmonary atelectasis and the characteristic clinical picture described above. On roentgen examination, a diffuse reticulogranular pattern and air bronchograms are observed. The increase in the phospholipid component of the surfactant with advancing gestational age forms the basis of the specific tests of pulmonary maturity (L/S ratio, phosphatidylglycerol (PG) determination, and FST).

The long suspected increase in the risk for RDS in IDMs has been examined and confirmed in a retrospective analysis by Robert et al (56). If other variables were excluded, including gestational age, delivery by cesarean section, presence of labor, birth weight, sex, Apgar score at five minutes, antepartum hemorrhage, presence of hydramnios, maternal anemia, and maternal age, the relative risk was 5.6% times higher in the IDM. This effect was especially evident in infants of gestational age ≤ 38 weeks. However, with improved obstetrical management, the frequency of RDS appears to be decreasing.

Recognition that RDS commonly occurs in the IDM led to evaluations of alternative diagnostic tests. In 1973, two years after initially reporting on the value of the L/S ratio in normal pregnancies, Gluck and Kulovich noted a delayed L/S maturation in patients with diabetes in White's classes A, B, and C, whereas an accelerated maturation was found in patients of classes D, E, and F (57). Indeed, when the L/S ratio equals 2.0, there may be an increased frequency of "false positives" in all diabetic classes.

A diagnostic refinement is provided by quantitative chromotographic assays for phosphatidylinositol (PI) and PG. It has been shown that a low PG and a high PI are signs of possible RDS even when the L/S ratio is ≥ 2 (58).

The increase in surfactant production from dipalmitoyl lecithin may be related to the secretion of cortisol relative to that of insulin. Indeed, it has been shown that insulin inhibits the incorporation of choline into lecithin, even when cortisol is present (59), and the incorporation of glucose and fatty acid into phosphatidylcholine in fetal rabbit lung slices (60). Thus, endogenous insulin, known to be increased in the fetus of the poorly controlled pregnant diabetic woman, may play a role in delaying pulmonary maturation. Although the specific biochemical mechanisms are unclear, these studies correlate with the clinical situation in which pulmonary maturation is delayed and RDS is noted but the L/S ratio is ≥ 2.0.

Hypoglycemia

A rapid fall in plasma glucose concentration following delivery is characteristic of the IDM. Values less than 35 mg/dL in term infants and less than 25 mg/dL in preterm infants may occur within 30 minutes after clamping the umbilical vessels, may persist for 48 hours, or may develop 24 hours after birth. Factors that are known to influence the degree of hypoglycemia include prior maternal glucose homeostasis, and maternal glycemia during delivery (61). An inadequately controlled pregnant diabetic woman will have stimulated the fetal pancreas to synthesize excessive amounts of insulin, which may be readily released. Administration of intravenous dextrose during the intrapartum period, which results in maternal hyperglycemia (> 125 mg/dL), may further stimulate the fetal pancreas. Another factor that may contribute to the development of hypoglycemia is a defective maturation of the counterregulation by catecholamines, glucagon, and/or other hormones (33).

Insulin Counterregulation

Several groups of investigators have studied the epinephrine and norepinephrine response to hypoglycemia in IDMs, with inconsistent results. An early study involved 11 IDMs, two of whom had gestational diabetes, and ten infants of normal mothers. The urinary epinephrine and norepinephrine levels of the IDMs did not increase following an episode of severe maternal hypoglycemia, but did rise when the hypoglycemia was mild (26). From results of a similar investigation, Stern et al suggested that long-standing hypoglycemia in the infant would lead to adrenal medullary exhaustion, presumably secondary to poor control of maternal diabetes (62). This hypothesis was confirmed by the subsequent observation that the plasma glucose, free fatty acid, and insulin responses to exogenous epinephrine were appropriate in IDMs (63). A converse explanation was given by Young et al to explain the high plasma norepinephrine concentrations in IDMs whose degree of glycemic control was not reported except that some of the infants were borderline large for gestational age (64). They speculated that the IDM exposed to excessive quantities of glucose may be subject to chronic sympathoadrenal stimulation. Artel et al also found elevated levels of plasma epinephrine and norepinephrine in IDMs and considered them evidence of hypersecretion; they proposed that neonatal hypoglycemia might be secondary to adrenal exhaustion (65).

Broberger et al evaluated the sympathoadrenal activity in the first 12 hours after birth in infants of nine women with type I diabetes and 13 women with insulin-treated gestational diabetes. Failure to observe differences in plasma epinephrine and norepinephrine levels between IDMs and control infants was felt to be secondary to good metabolic control of the diabetic mother (66).

Recently, as part of our continuing investigation of neonatal glucose metabolism, we infused epinephrine (50 mg or 500 mg/kg/min) into newborn lambs and measured glucose turnover by means of 6-[^{3}H]-glucose. The newborn lamb showed a blunted response to the lower dose of infused epinephrine. We speculated that if a similar phenomenon could be demonstrated in the IDM, it could partially account for the observed hypoglycemia (67,68). However, these results have to be reconciled with those of Keenan et al (63) discussed above.

Most IDMs are asymptomatic even when profoundly hypoglycemic, perhaps thanks to adequate initial stores of glucagon. Even when signs and symptoms are present, they are not specific and include tachypnea, apnea, tremulousness, sweating, irritability, and seizures. Asymptomatic infants do not require parenteral treatment. Early feeding at three to four hours of age may, however, be beneficial if plasma glucose levels are not severely depressed. The best therapy is prevention and consists of rigid control of maternal blood glucose levels during pregnancy and delivery with measurements of glucose in the umbilical blood at the time of delivery. The plasma glucose of the infant should be measured by a rapid bedside technique ½, 2, and 4 hours after birth and before each feeding until stable. Abnormal values should be verified by more precise methods.

The symptomatic infant should receive an intravenous bolus of 0.25 g/kg of dextrose in a 25% solution administered over two to four minutes, followed by a continuous infusion at the rate of 4 to 6 mg/kg/min. Bolus injections alone without subsequent infusion will only cause reactive hypoglycemia and are contraindicated. Once the plasma glucose stabilizes above 45 mg/dL, the infusion may be gradually decreased while oral feeding is initiated or increased. If hypoglycemia persists, it may be necessary to increase the rate of glucose infusion 8 to 12 mg/kg/min or more.

Glucagon may be administered within 15 minutes of delivery to prevent hypoglycemia. However, since most infants are asymptomatic, this does not appear warranted, especially since glucagon may stimulate insulin release and thus exaggerate the tendency to hypoglycemia.

Prompt recognition and treatment of symptomatic infants is believed to minimize the sequelae of hypoglycemia, although no late central nervous system complications have been attributed to it (69). Whether the occasional delay in motor development or psychologic dysfunction observed after five years is related to early hypoglycemia is unclear.

Hypocalcemia and Hypomagnesemia

Hypocalcemia is another major metabolic derangement in the IDM (70). During a normal pregnancy, a relative state of maternal hyperparathyroidism increases calcium mobilization from the bone, thus compensating for the calcium transferred to the fetus. Indeed, the concentration of calcium in the fetal blood is generally higher than in the mother, and, consequently, the secretion of calcitonin is stimulated.

At birth a combination of high calcitonin levels and interruption of the maternal supply of calcium causes the serum calcium to fall. Hypocalcemia, in turn, sets in motion a parathyroid-hormone (PTH)-induced and 1,25 dihydroxyvitamin D-induced counterregulation. A defect in this homeostatic mechanism may be the reason for the hypocalcemia in infants who are born prematurely, who are asphyxiated, or who are born to diabetic mothers (71–74). Indeed, approximately 50% of the infants born to insulin-dependent diabetic women develop hypocalcemia ($\leq$ 7 mg/dL) during the first three days of life (70). This high incidence of hypocalcemia is not seen in infants of gestational diabetic women. Prematurity and asphyxia (both of which may be present in IDMs) do not appear to be independent pathogenetic factors. However, the frequency and severity of serum hypocalcemia are directly related to the severity of the diabetes and may be aggravated by neonatal asphyxia. It has been postulated that neonatal hyperphosphatemia may also be a contributing factor.

Failure of an appropriate rise in PTH concentration in response to hypocalcemia has been reported in hypocalcemic infants of insulin-dependent diabetic mothers (74). This lack of response may be the result of hypomagnesemia (1.5 mg/dL), which has been found in as many as 33% of IDMs and whose frequency and severity appear correlated not only with the magnesium concentration in the mother, but also with the maternal insulin requirements and with the amount of glucose administered intravenously to the infant (74).

Hypocalcemia and hypomagnesemia, which have clinical manifestations similar to those of hypoglycemia, must be considered and treated appropriately. Their potential long-term deleterious effects are unknown.

Hyperbilirubinemia and Erythremia

Hyperbilirubinemia is observed more frequently in the IDM than in the normal infant. Although several hypotheses have been suggested, its pathogenesis remains uncertain. Gestational age is an unlikely cause, since jaundice is more common in IDMs than in age-matched non-IDMs (75). The increased incidence of Coombs' positive ABO blood group incompatibility reported in some IDMs has not been confirmed (76). It has been suggested that hyperbilirubinemia may be the result of hemolysis with decreased red cell survival, although red cell life span, osmotic fragility, and deformability have not been found to be appreciably different in IDMs, nor have an increased umbilical cord bilirubin or an increased postnatal rate of hemoglobin decline been demonstrated. Recently, Peevy et al suggested that only macrosomic IDMs are at risk of hyperbilirubinemia and that an increased heme turnover is a significant factor in its pathogenesis (77). Another contributing factor could be a delayed clearance of bilirubin load (78,79).

The most important factor associated with hyperbilirubinemia in the IDM may well be erythremia. Venous hematocrits $\geq$ 65% have been observed in 20% to 40% of IDMs, sometimes associated with signs and symptoms such as the jitters, seizures, tachypnea, priapism, and oliguria. Therapy by partial exchange transfusion (10% to 15% of total blood volume) with plasmanate or 5% albumin through the umbilical vein brings about rapid resolution of the symptoms. The relationship of neonatal erythremia to maternal blood glucose control and/or other perinatal factors associated with diabetic pregnancy has not been studied.

Fetal hypoxia in IDMs may explain neonatal erythremia and hyperbilirubinemia. The umbilical cord levels of erythropoietin, a hormone whose production is stimulated by hypoxia, were found to be above the narrow normal range in one third of 61 IDMs (80). Moreover, this increase was correlated with neonatal hyperinsulinemia. Normal fetal monkeys made hyperinsulinemic in the last third of gestation had markedly elevated plasma erythropoietin levels as well as other evidence of increased fetal erythropoiesis, such as elevated reticulocyte counts (81). In addition, chronic hyperglycemia in fetal sheep, achieved by infusing glucose through an implanted intravenous catheter, resulted in increased oxygen consumption and decreased distal aortic arterial oxygen content (82).

Finally, it has been suggested that IDMs may suffer ineffective erythropoiesis, defined as the failure to release erythrocytes from erythropoietic organs. Support for this hypothesis comes from the observation that in IDMs the excretion of carbon monoxide derived from heme metabolism is greater in IDMs than in normal infants matched for gestational age (78,79). Hemoglobin levels were not significantly higher in the IDM, nor was hemolysis, as evaluated by Coombs' positive blood group incompatibility. A possibly related observation is the delay in the fetal globin switch in IDMs reported by Perrine et al (83).

Renal Vein Thrombosis

Renal vein thrombosis is a rare but severe life-threatening occurrence in the perinatal period (84). It is more frequently observed in IDMs than in normal infants. Although Pedersen failed to mention this condition in his monograph, one postmortem survey revealed that five of the 16 cases of neonatal renal vein thrombosis had occurred in IDMs (85) and seven others in infants born to mothers without known diabetes but with fetal macrosomia and pancreatic β-cell hypertrophy and hyperplasia. A case of IDM with a nearly totally occlusive thrombosis of the umbilical vein has also been reported (86).

The pathogenesis of this lesion is obscure, although erythremia appears to be a probable factor. Sludging of blood combined with reduction of cardiac output, possibly aggravated by diabetic cardiomyopathy, may be a contributing factor. Stuart et al suggested that an increased production of platelet endoperoxides in the IDM may upset the normal balance between proaggregatory (platelet) and antiaggregatory (vascular) prostaglandins, favoring the development of thrombosis (87). Whatever the mechanism of thrombosis, the reasons for its predilection in the renal vein is obscure. Birth trauma is an unlikely initiating factor, since this lesion has been observed in stillborns as well as in IDMs delivered by cesarean section. In one case, venous thrombosis was observed in the stillborn infant of a diabetic mother who had received oxytocin for the induction of labor (88).

In the liveborn infant, the salient diagnostic features of renal vein thrombosis are hematuria and the presence of a flank mass. Therapy requires careful maintenance of fluid and electrolyte balance and the correction of erythremia by plasma exchange. Nephrectomy should be considered, while the role of heparinization remains controversial.

Long-Term Prognosis and Follow-up

The previous discussion has dealt only with problems encountered during the neonatal period. Of equal concern and perhaps of greater ultimate importance are the long-term effects of maternal diabetes on the growth, physical, psychosocial, and intellectual development of the offspring and of developing diabetes. Here, again, perhaps the most important factor influencing long-term prognosis is the management of the pregnant diabetic woman and her infant. If, indeed, many of the deleterious effects of diabetes in pregnancy can be avoided by correcting the metabolic status of the pregnant woman and in her conceptus, the poor prognosis reported in previous retrospective studies should not show up in future prospective evaluations.

There are few prospective studies of growth and development of the IDM. Farquhar's analysis of 231 of a group of 320 infants is significant because it revealed that more children up to 15 years of age fell below the third percentile for height than exceeded the 97th percentile (21 versus 5) (89). By contrast, an equal number of children were overweight or underweight, although examination of the weight-to-height indices suggested that excessive weight was more common than low weight. Farquhar suggested that this may represent a "return to obesity" noted at birth. In another study Bibergeil noted that height was elevated in 16.7% but below normal in 9.3% and that children whose neonatal weight was greater than 4 kg were significantly taller and heavier when they reached school age (90). Somatic growth of children of diabetic mothers was studied also by Vohr et al (91), who suggested that macrosomia in the IDM may be a harbinger of obesity, since eight of 19 offspring of diabetic women who had been large for gestational age at birth, but only one of 14 who had not, were obese at age 7.

It is recognized that congenital malformations may in themselves represent neuropsychologic handicaps. Nevertheless, Yssing found that 36% of 265 children born to diabetic mothers had evidence of cerebral dysfunction or related conditions (92). Cerebral palsy and epilepsy were found to be three to five times higher than in the normal population, but there was no difference in the frequency of mental retardation. When present, the difficulties seemed to be related to extreme age of the mother, severity of diabetes, low birth weight for gestational age, or complications during pregnancy.

Psychologic evaluation of children at 1, 3, and 5 years of age suggested that at ages 3 and 5 the IDM is more vulnerable to intellectual impairment, especially if born small for gestational age or if the pregnancy had been complicated by acetonuria (93).

On the other hand, Persson et al found no evidence that asymptomatic neonatal hypoglycemia per se leads to intellectual impairment by 5 years of age (69).

The question whether the IDM has an increased likelihood of becoming diabetic has been analysed and reviewed. If one parent has insulin-dependent diabetes mellitus, the empiric risk of the offspring developing insulin-dependent diabetes mellitus is 1% to 5% (94). Although family aggregates exist, a simple mode of inheritance is inconsistent with the reported data (95), and the suggestion has been made that a polygenic multifactorial model best explains the reported observations (94). Thus, it appears that the infant born to a parent with diabetes is at risk for developing the disease.

Conclusion

Although survival, morbidity, and development are constantly improving, infants born to diabetic mothers remain a high-risk population, and much work remains to be done until the underlying pathophysiology is understood. Optimal results are obtained when meticulous medical-obstetric care throughout pregnancy is combined with expert neonatal supervision. Thus, these high-risk patients should be delivered in tertiary care centers providing specialized management.

Acknowledgment. This chapter was supported in part by the National Institute of Health-National Institute of Child Health and Human Development (NIH-NICHHD) 1-550 HD 11343. During the period of the studies reported here, Dr. Cowett was the recipient of an RCDA 1-KO4 HD 00308 from the NIH-NICHHD.

References

1. Wolfe RR, Allsop J, Burke JF (1979) Glucose metabolism in man: Responses to intravenous glucose. Metab Clin Exp 28:210–220.

2. Cowett RM (1985) Pathophysiology, Diagnosis and Management of Glucose Homeostasis in the Neonate, in Lockhart J (ed): Clinical Problems in Pediatrics. Yearbook, Chicago, pp 1–43.
3. Schwartz R, Cowett RM, Widness JA (1980) Infants of Diabetic Mothers, in Brodoff BN, Bleicher SJ (eds): Diabetes Mellitus and Obesity. Williams & Wilkins Company, Baltimore, pp 601–610.
4. Cowett RM, Schwartz R (1982) The infant of the diabetic mother, in Oh W (ed): Symposium on the Newborn. Pediatr Clin North Am, 29:1213–1231.
5. Cornblath M, Schwartz R (1976) Disorders of Carbohydrate Metabolism in Infancy, ed 2. WB Saunders, Philadelphia, pp 115–154.
6. Jovanovic L, Druzin M, Peterson CM (1980) Effects of euglycemia on the outcome of pregnancy in insulin-dependent diabetic women as compared with normal control subjects. Am J Med 68:105–112.
7. Kitzmiller JL, Cloherty JP, Younger MD, et al (1978) Diabetic pregnancy and perinatal morbidity. Am J Obstet Gynecol 131:560–568.
8. Pedersen J, Molsted-Pedersen L, Andersen B (1974) Assessors of fetal perinatal mortality in diabetic pregnancy. Analyses of 1332 pregnancies in the Copenhagen series 1946–1972. Diabetes 23:302–305.
9. Hare JW, White P (1980) Gestational diabetes and the White classification. Diabetes Care 3:394.
10. Pollak A, Brehm R, Havelec L, et al (1981) Total glycosylated hemoglobin in mothers of large for gestational age infants: A postpartum test for undetected maternal diabetes? Biol Neonate 40:129–135.
11. Widness JA, Schwartz HC, Zeller WP, et al (1981) Glycohemoglobin in postpartum women. Obstet Gynecol 57:414–421.
12. Teramo K, Kuusisto AN, Raivio KO (1979) Perinatal outcome of insulin-dependent diabetic pregnancies. Ann Clin Res 11:146–155.
13. Jerwell J, Bjerkedal T, Moe N (1980) Outcome of pregnancies in diabetic mothers in Norway 1967–1976. Diabetologia, 18:131–134.
14. Artal R, Golde SH, Dorey F, et al (1983) The effect of plasma glucose variability on neonatal outcome in the pregnant diabetic patient. Am J Obstet Gynecol 147:537–541.
15. Jovanovic R, Jovanovic L (1984) Obstetric management when normoglycemia is maintained in diabetic women with vascular compromise. Am J Obstet Gynecol 149:617–623.
16. Coustan DR, Imarah J (1984) Prophylactic insulin treatment of gestational diabetes reduces the incidence of macrosomia, operative delivery, and birth trauma. Am J Obstet Gynecol 150:836–842.
17. Pedersen J (1977) The pregnant diabetic and her newborn, ed 2. Munksgaard International Publishers Ltd., Copenhagen, pp 1–280.
18. Naeye RL (1965) Infants of diabetic mothers: A quantitative morphologic study. Pediatr 35:980–988.
19. Susa JB, McCormick KL, Widness JA, et al (1979) Chronic hyperinsulinemia in the fetal rhesus monkey. Effects on fetal growth and composition. Diabetes 28:1058–1063.
20. Block MD, Pildes RS, Mossabhou NA, et al (1974) C-peptide immunoreactivity (CRP): A new method for studying infants of insulin-treated diabetic mothers. Pediatrics 53:923–928.
21. King KC, Adam PAJ, Yamaguchi K, et al (1974) Insulin response to arginine

in normal newborn infants and infants of diabetic mothers. Diabetes, 23:816–820.
22. Pildes RS, Hart RJ, Warner R, et al (1969) Plasma insulin response during oral glucose tolerance tests in newborns of normal and gestational diabetic mothers. Pediatrics 44:76–82.
23. Isles PE, Dickson M, Farquhar JW (1968) Glucose intolerance and plasma insulin in newborn infants of normal and diabetic mothers. Pediatr Res 2:198–208.
24. Adam PAJ, King KC, Schwartz R (1968) Model for investigation of intractable hypoglycemia. Insulin glucose interrelationships during steady state infusion. Pediatrics 41:91–105.
25. King KC, Adam PAJ, Clements GA, et al (1969) Infants of diabetic mothers: Attenuated glucose uptake without hyperinsulinemia during continuous glucose infusions. Pediatrics 44:381–392.
26. Light IJ, Sutherland JM, Loggie JM, et al (1967) Impaired epinephrine release in hypoglycemic infants of diabetic mothers. N Engl J Med 277:394–398.
27. Bloom SR, Johnston DT (1972) Failure of glucagon release in infants of diabetic mothers. Br Med J 4:453–454.
28. Kaplan SA, Neufeld ND, Lippe BM, et al (1979) Maternal diabetes and the development of the insulin receptor, in Merkatz IR, Adam PAJ (eds): The diabetic pregnancy. A perinatal perspective. Grune & Stratton, New York, pp 169–173.
29. Kalhan SC, Savin SM, Adam PAJ (1977) Attenuated glucose production rate in newborn infants of insulin-dependent diabetic mothers. N Engl J Med 296:375–376.
30. King KC, Tserng KY, Kalhan SC (1982) Regulation of glucose production in newborn infants of diabetic mothers. Pediatr Res 16:608–612.
31. Cowett RM, Susa JB, Giletti B, et al (1980) Variability of endogenous glucose production in infants of insulin dependent diabetic mothers. Pediatr Res 14:570.
32. Cowett RM, Susa JB, Gilette B, et al (1983) Glucose kinetics in infants of diabetic mothers. Am J Obstet Gynecol 146:781–786.
33. Cowett RM, Oh W, Schwartz J, et al (1983) Persistent glucose production during glucose infusion in the neonate. J Clin Invest 71:467–473.
34. Widness JA, Cowett RM, Coustan DR, et al (1985) Neonatal morbidities in infants of mothers with glucose intolerance in pregnancy. Diabetes 34 [Suppl 2]: 61–65.
35. Freinkel N (1980) Of pregnancy and progeny, Banting Lecture, Diabetes 29:1023–1035.
36. Milner RDG (1979) Amino acids and beta cell growth in structure and function in Merkatz IR, Adam PAJ (eds): The Diabetic Pregnancy. A Perinatal Perspective. Grune & Stratton, New York, pp 145–153.
37. Kucera J (1971) Rate and type of congenital anomalies among offspring of diabetic women. J Reprod Med 7:61–70.
38. Pedersen LM, Tygstrup I, Pedersen J (1964) Congenital malformations in newborn infants of diabetic women. Correlation with maternal diabetic vascular complication. Lancet 1:1124–1126.
39. Roversi GD, Gugiulo M, Nicolini U, et al (1979) A new approach to the treatment of diabetic pregnant women. Am J Obstet Gynecol 135:567–576.
40. Neave C (1984) Congenital malformation in offspring of diabetics. Perspect Pediatr Pathol 8:213–222.

41. Fuhrmann K, Reiher H, Semmler K, et al (1983) Prevention of congenital malformations in infants of insulin dependent diabetic mothers. Diabetes Care 6:219–223.
42. Miller E, Hare JW, Cloherty JP, et al (1981) Elevated maternal hemoglobin A_{1c} in early pregnancy and major congenital anomalies in infants of diabetic mothers. N Engl J Med 304:1331–1134.
43. Goldman JA, Dicker D, Feldberg D, et al (1986) Pregnancy outcome in patients with insulin dependent diabetes mellitus with preconceptual diabetes control: A comparative study. Am J Obstet Gynecol 155:293–297.
44. Ballard JL, Holroyde J, Tsang RC, et al (1984) High malformation rates and decreased mortality in infants of diabetic mothers managed after the first trimester (1956–1978). Am J Obstet Gynecol 148:111–118.
45. Landauer W (1945) Rumplessness in chicken embryos produced by the injection of insulin and other chemicals. J Exp Zool 98:65–77.
46. Adam PAJ, Teramo K, Raiha N, et al (1969) Human fetal insulin metabolism early in gestation. Diabetes 18:409–416.
47. Widness JA, Goldman AS, Susa JB, et al (1983) Impermeability of the rat placenta to insulin during organogenesis. Teratology 28:327–332.
48. Davis WS, Allen RP, Favara BE, et al (1974) Neonatal small left colon syndrome. Am J Roent Rad Therap Nucl Med 120:327–329.
49. Way GL, Wolfe RR, Eshughpour E, et al (1979) The natural history of hypertrophic cardiomyopathy in infants of diabetic mothers. J Pediatr 95:1020–1025.
50. Mace S, Hirschfeld SS, Riggs T, et al (1979) Echocardiographic abnormalities in infants of diabetic mothers. J Pediatr 95:1013–1019.
51. Breitweser JA, Mayer RA, Sperling MA, et al (1980) Cardiac septal hypertrophy in hyperinsulinemic infants. J Pediatr 96:535–539.
52. Halliday HL (1981) Hypertrophic cardiomyopathy in infants or poorly controlled diabetic mothers. Arch Dis Child 56:258–263.
53. Molsted-Pedersen L, Pedersen JF (1985) Congenital malformations in diabetic pregnancies. Acta Paediatr Scand [Suppl] 32:79–84.
54. Cruz AC, Buhi WC, Birk SA, et al (1976) Respiratory distress syndrome with mature lecithin/sphingomyelin ratios, diabetes mellitus and low Apgar scores. Am J Obstet Gynecol 126:78–82.
55. Hsi Ac, Davis DJ, Sherman FC (1985) Neonatal gangrene in the newborn infant of a diabetic mother. J Pediatr Orthop 5:358–360.
56. Robert MD, Nel RK, Hubbell JP, et al (1976) Association between maternal diabetes and the respiratory distress syndrome in the newborn. N Engl J Med 294:357–360.
57. Gluck L, Kulovich MV (1973) Lecithin/sphingomyelin ratios in amniotic fluid in normal and abnormal pregnancies. Am J Obstet Gynecol 115:539–546.
58. Hallman M, Teramo K (1979) Amniotic fluid phospholipid profile as a predictor of fetal maturity in diabetic pregnancies. Obstet Gynecol 54:703–707.
59. Smith BT, Giroud CJP, Robert M, et al (1975) Insulin antagonism of cortisol action on lecithin synthesis by cultured fetal lung cells. J Pediatr 87:953–955.
60. Neufeld ND, Sevanian A, Barrett CT, et al (1979) Inhibition of surfactant production by insulin in fetal rabbit lung slices. Pediatr Res 13:752–754.
61. Cowett RM, Stern L (1987) Carbohydrate homeostasis in the fetus and newborn. Avery G (ed), Neonatology, Pathophysiology and Management of the Newborn. Lippincott & Co, Philadelphia, pp 691–709.

62. Stern L, Ramos A, Leduc J (1968) Urinary catecholamine excretion in infants of diabetic mothers. Pediatrics 42:598–605.
63. Keenan WJ, Light IJ, Sutherland JM (1972) Effects of exogenous epinephrine on glucose and insulin levels in infants of diabetic mothers. Biol Neonate 21:44–53.
64. Young BJ, Cohen WR, Rappaport EB, et al (1979) High plasma norepinephrine concentrations at birth in infants of diabetic mothers. Diabetes 28:697–699.
65. Artel R, Platt LD, Kammula RK, et al (1982) Sympatho-adrenal activity in infants of diabetic mothers. Am J Obstet Gynecol 142:436–439.
66. Broberger U, Hansson U, Lagercrantz H, et al (1984) Sympatho-adrenal activity and metabolic adjustment during the first 12 hours after birth in infants of diabetic mothers. Acta Pediatr Scand 73:620–625.
67. Cowett RM (1985) Decreased neonatal responsiveness to catecholamines: Effect on glucose kinetics. Pediatr Res 19:152A.
68. Cowett RM (1985) Alpha adrenergic stimulate neonatal glucose production less than beta adrenergic. Pediatr Res 19:311A.
69. Persson B, Gentz J, Lunell NO (1978) Diabetes in pregnancy, in Scarpelli EM, Cosmi EV (eds): Reviews in Perinatal Medicine, vol 2. Raven Press, New York, pp 1–53.
70. Tsang RC, Brown DR, Steinchen JJ (1979) Diabetes and calcium disturbances in infants of diabetic mothers in Merkatz IR, Adam PAJ (eds): The Diabetic Pregnancy. A Perinatal Perspective. Grune & Stratton, New York, pp 207–225.
71. Tsang RC, Kleinman L, Sutherland JM (1972) Hypocalcemia in infants of diabetic mothers: Studies in Ca, P and Mg Metabolism and in parathyroid hormone responsiveness. J Pediatr 80:384–355.
72. Tsang RC, Light IJ, Sutherland JM, et al (1973) Possible pathogenetic factors in neonatal hypocalcemia of prematurity. J Pediatric 82:423–429.
73. Tsang RC, Chen I, Atkinson W, et al (1974) Neonatal hypocalcemia in birth asphyxia. J Pediatr 84:428–433.
74. Noguchi A, Erin M, Tsang RC (1980) Parathyroid hormone in hypocalcemic and normocalcemic infants of diabetic mothers. J Pediatr 97:112–114.
75. Taylor PM, Wolfson J, Bright NH, et al (1963) Hyperbilirubinemia in infants of diabetic mothers. Biol Neonate 5:289.
76. Zetterstrom R, Strindberg B, Arnhold RG (1958) Hyperbilirubinemia in ABO hemolytic disease in newborn infants of diabetic mothers. Acta Paediatr 47:238.
77. Peevy KJ, Landaw SA, Gross SA (1980) Hyperbilirubinemia in infants of diabetic mothers. Pediatrics 66:417–419.
78. Stevenson DF, Ostrander CR, Cohen RS, et al (1981) Pulmonary excretion of carbon monoxide in the human infant as an index of bilirubin production. Eur J Pediatr 137:255–259.
79. Stevenson DR, Ostrander CR, Hopper AO, et al (1981) Pulmonary excretion of carbon monoxide as an index of bilirubin production. IIa. Evidence for possible delayed clearance of bilirubin in infants of diabetic mothers. J Pediatr 98:822–824.
80. Widness JA, Susa J, Garcia JF, et al (1981) Increased erythropoiesis and elevated erythropoietin in infants born to diabetic mothers and in hyperinsulinemic rhesus fetuses. J Clin Invest 67:637–642.
81. Carson BS, Philipps AF, Simmons MA, et al (1980) Effects of a sustained

insulin infusion upon glucose uptake and oxygenation of the ovine fetus. Pediatr Res 14:147–152.

82. Philipps AF, Widness JA, Garcia JF, et al (1982) Erythropoietin elevation in the chronically hyperglycemic fetal lamb. Proc Soc Exp Biol Med 170:42–47.

83. Perrine SP, Greene MF, Faller DV (1985) Delay in the fetal globin switch in infants of diabetic mothers. N Engl J Med 312:334–338.

84. Avery ME, Oppenheimer EH, Gordon HH (1957) Renal vein thrombosis in newborn infants of diabetic mothers. N Engl J Med 265:1134–1138.

85. Takeuchi A, Benirschke K (1961) Renal vein thrombosis of the newborn and its relation to maternal diabetes. Biol Neonate 3:237.

86. Fritz MA, Christopher CR (1981) Umbilical vein thrombosis and maternal diabetes mellitus. J Reprod Med 26:320–323.

87. Stuart MJ, Sunderji-Shirazali G, Allen JB (1981) Decreased prostacyclin production in the infant of the diabetic mother. J Lab Clin Med 98:412–416.

88. Al-Samarrai SF, Kato A, Urano Y (1984) Renal vein thrombosis in stillborn infants of diabetic mothers. Acta Pathol Jpn 34:1411–1447.

89. Farquhar JW (1969) Prognosis for babies born to diabetic mothers in Edinburgh. Arch Dis Child 44:36–47.

90. Bibergeil H, Bodel E, Amendt P (1975) Diabetes and Pregnancy: Early and late prognoses of children of diabetic mothers, in Camerini-Davalos RA, Cole HS (eds): Early Diabetes in Early Life. Academic Press, New York, pp 427–434.

91. Vohr BR, Lipsitt LP, Oh W (1980) Somatic growth of children of diabetic mothers with reference to birth size. J Pediatr 97:196–199.

92. Yssing M (1975) Long-term prognosis of children born to mothers diabetic when pregnant in Camerini-Davalos RA, Cole HS (eds): Early Diabetes in Early-Life. Academic Press, New York, pp 575–586.

93. Stehbens JA, Baker GL, Kitchell M (1977) Outcome at ages 1, 3, and 5 years of children born to diabetic women. Am J Obstet Gynecol 127:408–413.

94. Anderson CE, Rotter JI, Rimoin DL (1981) Genetics of diabetes mellitus, in Rifkin H, Raskin P (eds): Diabetes Mellitus, vol V. F Brady, Annapolis, Maryland, p 79.

95. Simpson JL (1979) Genetics of diabetes mellitus and anomalies in offspring of diabetic mothers in Merkatz IR, Adam PAJ (eds): The Diabetic Pregnancy. A Perinatal Perspective. Grune & Stratton, New York, pp 249–260.

11
Long-Term Outlook for the Offspring of the Diabetic Woman

KATHRYN R. SLAINE, PETER H. BENNETT, AND DAVID J. PETTITT

Morphologically and metabolically, infants of diabetic mothers differ from infants of nondiabetic mothers. At birth many of these infants are macrosomic and have hypertrophic, hyperplastic pancreatic islet cells. On long-term follow-up, the offspring of diabetic women tend to be obese and to have abnormal glucose tolerance.

Obesity in Infants of Diabetic Mothers

Adipocyte Development

Many factors operating in utero, including genetic makeup, maternal obesity, maternal weight change during gestation, and maternal endocrine status, have been found to modify adipose tissue growth resulting in alterations of either fat-cell size or fat cell number (1–9). Postnatally, hyperphagia and high-fat diets are also important factors in fat-cell development, with saturated fats leading to an increase in both fat-cell size and number while unsaturated fats in the diet lead to an increase in size only (1). Current knowledge of adipocyte development in children is derived from a number of sources, including cell culture studies, adipose tissue biopsies, and epidemiologic data.

Adipocyte transplantation studies, in which adipocytes from genetically obese mice were transplanted into genetically lean mice and vice versa, have provided evidence of extracellular factors that control fat-cell size and fatty-acid composition (2). The adipocytes from genetically obese mice normalized in both size and fatty-acid composition after transplantation to lean mice, and, conversely, normal size adipocytes from lean animals transplanted into obese animals enlarged to a size similar to that of the host's adipocytes. These observations suggest that some extracellular, possibly endocrine, factor is important in regulating lipolysis and lipogenesis in the adipose tissue of genetically obese mice.

Growth of the preadipocyte and differentiation into the mature adipocyte can be observed in tissue culture, and the role of hormones in proliferation of the preadipocyte can be tested. Several investigators (3–8) have evaluated the effect of various hormones on the differentiation of preadipocytes into the mature adipocytes in animal cell culture. Growth hormone influences proliferation of the preadipocytes in cell culture (3), although this has not been shown in vivo, and 17 β-estradiol stimulates multiplication of adipocyte precursors in culture (4). The extracts of some organs, such as the pituitary gland, have both stimulatory and inhibitory activity (5), stimulation being apparent only at concentrations too low for the inhibitors to be active. Insulin administration during early life in animals influences the size but not the number of adipocytes; but in tissue culture at very high concentrations, insulin is a potent inducer of preadipocyte differentiation (6). A number of other hormones and drugs affect the rate of accumulation of triglyceride but have little or no effect on conversion of preadipocytes to adipocytes (7). Kuri-Harcuch et al (8) collected serum from pregnant women at various gestational ages as well as from the umbilical cord of infants at delivery and examined the effect of the serum on cell differentiation in an established mouse preadipocyte line. Adipocyte differentiation was significantly higher when incubated with serum collected from the mother or from cord blood after 33 weeks of gestation than with cord blood or maternal serum collected before that time or from adult males. By two days after delivery, adipogenic activity in the mothers had decreased to normal levels. Amniotic fluid obtained by amniocentesis from women between 30 and 36 weeks of gestation produced a much lower rate of differentiation of adipocyte tissue than fetal or maternal serum. After 33 weeks of gestation, the mother or infant or both may secrete an adipogenic factor, which stimulates adipocyte differentiation. Such a substance, however, remains to be identified.

Adipocyte Development in Normal Children

Despite studies by a number of investigators (10–16), it is still not certain exactly when and how body-fat growth occurs in humans. The matter has been reviewed in detail by Bonnet and Rocour-Brumioul (10) and can be summarized as follows. Most normal growth in fat-cell size occurs during the last month or two of fetal development and ends before 2 years of age. Subsequently, in normal children adipocyte size remains relatively constant (11). The number of adipocytes also increases most rapidly during late gestation and early infancy and remains constant until adolescence, when it increases again in coincidence with the onset of puberty in boys and prepuberty in girls (12). After adolescence there is little change in cell number. The intrauterine hormonal influences on adipocyte development have been examined by Enzi, et al (13), who looked at the relationships between maternal nutritional and hormonal factors and newborn body-fat mass. They found no correlation between either insulin or growth hormone in the mother and body-fat mass, fat-cell weight, or fat-cell number in the newborn. However, maternal glucose concentrations during an oral glucose tolerance test were correlated with neonatal body fat mass. Neonatal plasma insulin concentrations correlated with body-fat mass and fat-cell weight, but not with fat-cell number.

Evidence that patterns of obesity may be inherited comes from adoption and from twin studies (17–21). Adoption studies have shown a correlation between body habitus of offspring and their biologic parents while no correlation has been found between the body habitus of adoptees and their adoptive parents (17,18). During infancy, however, children cared for by obese foster mothers have a tendency, albeit not a statistically significant one, to be heavier than those cared for by nonobese foster mothers (19). Genetics, therefore, appears to have a strong influence on determining obesity, while environment, at least after the time of adoption, has little if any influence. A study of identical twins suggested that the changes in body fat that occurred during a 3-week period of overfeeding had a genetic basis (20). Börjeson (21), in a study of single siblings and of monozygotic and dizygotic twins, found that single siblings and fraternal twins had much greater variability in the amount of subcutaneous fat than did the monozygotic twins. He also concluded that heredity was the major determinant of obesity and that the environmental conditions did not cause obesity before the age of 7 years. On the other hand, the intrauterine environment also appears to have an effect on subsequent adiposity. Ginsberg-Fellner (22) evaluated the growth of the adipose tissue in 21 sets of twins. Identical twins with similar birth weights who were raised in the same environment had similar weights and adipose cell numbers in childhood. Identical twins discordant for birth weight, on the other hand, were discordant for adipose cell number and childhood weight, even if they were raised in the same environment. This discordance cannot be genetic, and it is assumed that intrauterine nutrition is largely responsible for determining birth weight. There was little similarity in obesity or adipose cell number between fraternal twins. Thus, it appears that discordance either in genetic makeup or in intrauterine experience may result in discordance of subsequent adiposity.

Maternal weight and weight change during gestation have been shown to have an effect on fetal adiposity. Both obesity and weight gain in the mother are associated with overweight in the newborn and are correlated with total-body-fat mass (14,23,24). No correlation, however, was shown between prepregnancy weight and fat-cell volume in the newborn.

The Macrosomic Infant

Perinatal difficulties, such as asphyxia neonatorum and birth trauma, which are associated with macrosomia, make fetal size of particular interest to the clinician. Macrosomic infants of diabetic women are heavier, have larger head circumferences, and a greater amount of subcutaneous fat than infants of nondiabetic mothers (25,26). Enzi et al (27) compared infants of women with gestational or insulin-dependent diabetes with infants of nondiabetic women and found that the infants of both gestational diabetic mothers and of mothers with insulin-dependent diabetes had an increased skinfold thickness and body-fat mass compared with controls. Length at birth is not uniformly increased, as some investigators found that the macrosomic infants of diabetic women were longer and other investigators found them to be shorter than average (28,29).

Long-Term Follow-up of Macrosomic Infants

In general, no correlation has been found between relative body size measured at birth or during early infancy and obesity during childhood and adolescence (30–32). There are some reports that most individuals who developed obesity in the first few years of life had been among the heaviest at birth (23,33), but on long-term follow-up, even infants whose birth weights were more than two standard deviations above the mean were not obese as adults (32).

The Effect of Maternal Diabetes on the Development of the Infant's Adipose Tissue

The macrosomic infant of a diabetic woman, because of the exposure to high concentrations of glucose during the third trimester of pregnancy, has big fat cells and a large fat mass with large skinfold thicknesses. There is a direct correlation between these characteristics and the diabetic mother's fasting blood glucose concentration (34).

Infants of gestational diabetic mothers and of obese nondiabetic mothers were examined at birth and followed for the first year of life with measurements of body-fat mass, skinfold thickness, and body weight. The infants of gestational diabetic mothers were heavier and had a larger adipocyte size than infants of nondiabetic mothers at birth. These differences did not persist and no correlation was found between the high birth weight and body-fat mass, sum of skinfold thickness, or body weight at 6 months of age (27). Björntorp et al. (32) examined the effects of maternal diabetes on adipose tissue cellularity in the offspring by following infants who were large for gestational age at birth. Hypercellularity was present in infants of women with gestational diabetes by 1 month of age and continued to increase with advancing age. Percent body weight of these infants increased after 2 years of age. In contrast, infants of mothers with type I diabetes did not exhibit adipose hypercellularity nor an increase in mean body weight until after their second birthday. However, as adolescents

TABLE 11.1. Adipose tissue cellularity in offspring of diabetic and nondiabetic women.

Maternal diabetes status	(n)	Adipose cell number at 1–17 months	Increased number 4–10 months later
Diabetic	(15)	5.3×10^9 Adipocytes	5/6
Nondiabetic	(10)	3.3×10^9 Adipocytes	0/2

Data from Ginsberg-Fellner F, Knittle JL (35).

and young adults, these offspring had neither increased amounts of body fat nor increased number or size of fat cells. Ginsberg-Fellner (22,35) also examined infants of nondiabetic women and of women with insulin-dependent and gestational diabetes. She found that infants of women with gestational diabetes and of those with insulin-dependent diabetes had increased numbers of fat cells compared with offspring of nondiabetic women. Adipose tissue hypercellularity was present in infants of gestational diabetic mothers by 1 month of age and continued to increase with advancing age (Table 11.1). Percent body weight of these infants, however, did not increase until after 2 years of age, although by age 7 years, 21 of the 23 children were obese. Adipose cell size also increased significantly during the first 7 years of life.

Abbott et al (36), on the other hand, found no difference between offspring of women with abnormal glucose tolerance during pregnancy, and of women who developed glucose intolerance only after pregnancy. They examined 9- and 10-year-old Pima Indian children who were born either to mothers with normal glucose tolerance during pregnancy but who later developed abnormal glucose tolerance, or to mothers who developed impaired glucose tolerance before or during pregnancy. No difference in body-fat mass, fat-free mass, or abdominal or gluteal adipocyte size was found between these groups (Table 11.2). However, in this study offspring of intolerant and preintolerant women were selected so as to be similar in height and weight, a method that may have led to the selection of children with similar fat-cell sizes.

TABLE 11.2. Abdominal and gluteal adipose cell sizes in the offspring of normal women and women with glucose intolerance during pregnancy (values are mean ± SE).

Group	Abdominal cell size (μg lipid/cell)	Gluteal cell size (μg lipid/cell)
Glucose intolerant pregnancy	0.60 + 0.05	0.69 + 0.03
Glucose tolerance pregnancy	0.62 + 0.05	0.68 + 0.04

From Abbott WGH et al (36). Reproduced with permission from the American Diabetes Association, Inc.

Growth Patterns of Infants of Diabetic Mothers

Evidence suggests that the intrauterine environment plays a role in the development of heavy-for-height children. In most studies that have examined growth patterns in childhood and adolescence, the children of women with diabetes have been found to be taller and heavier than expected from standard height and weight charts (37–39). Some studies, however, have found that the height or weight of children of diabetic mothers did not deviate significantly from the normal standards (40–42). Farquhar (43), in fact, noted that heights were on the short side; since these infants had a normal weight distribution, the weight/height ratio was larger than expected. There was some correlation between being overweight at birth and being overweight later in life. Infants who were greater than 150% of desirable weight at birth tended to have a weight-to-height ratio greater than 1.25 times the standard during childhood and adolescence (44).

Hagbard et al (45) examined children of diabetic and prediabetic mothers. The children of diabetic mothers were shorter and heavier than normals, while the offspring of prediabetic women were not different from normal. White et al (37) found that the sons and daughters of diabetic mothers were heavier than those of diabetic fathers. Vohr et al (46) examined and compared infants of mothers with gestational, type I, and type II diabetes and matched controls and found that macrosomic infants were born to nonobese diabetic mothers, but not to nonobese nondiabetic mothers. Macrosomic infants were also more commonly born to obese women if they had diabetes than if they did not. These macrosomic infants of diabetic women were more likely to be obese in childhood and adolescence than were normal birth weight infants (Table 11.3). Few offspring of nondiabetic women were obese when examined at age seven.

The Pima Indians of the Gila River Indian Community are examined

TABLE 11.3. Obesity at age 7 years and during adolescence in offspring of large-for-gestational age (LGA) and normal birth weight offspring of diabetic women and of controls at age 7 years. (Number of obese children followed by total in sample).

Maternal diabetes status	Birth weight	Age at examination	
		7 years	12–17 years
Diabetic	Normal	1 (14)	1 (13)
	LGA	8 (19)	6 (15)
Control	Normal	1 (26)	
	LGA	0 (4)	

Data from Vohr BR, et al (46).

periodically and pregnant women are given an oral glucose tolerance test after the 24th week of gestation. Mothers can therefore be classified as diabetic or nondiabetic during the pregnancy, or as prediabetic if they are nondiabetic during the pregnancy but develop diabetes at a later date (47).

Maternal diabetes is a risk factor for childhood obesity that is present by 5 to 9 years of age and persists to at least age 19 years (Figure 11.1). This relationship is not altered by maternal obesity although by the time the offspring reach the age of 15 to 19 years, an association between maternal obesity and obesity in offspring of nondiabetic and of prediabetic women appears to develop. Children of mothers with impaired glucose tolerance during pregnancy have a higher mean percent ideal weight than children of mothers with normal glucose tolerance, but a lower percent ideal weight than offspring of diabetic women (48). There was no difference in relative weight between the children of prediabetic and nondiabetic mothers. Figure 11.2 shows the direct relationship between mean percent desirable weight in the offspring and maternal glucose concentration during the pregnancy among women with no prior history of diabetes. Even children of diabetic mothers who were of normal weight at birth had a higher relative weight by age 5 to 9 years than the normal birth weight children of nondiabetic and prediabetic mothers, and this effect persisted to age 15 to 19 years (49).

Thus, the Pima experience suggests that the diabetic intrauterine environment is a causative factor of long-term obesity in the offspring. These

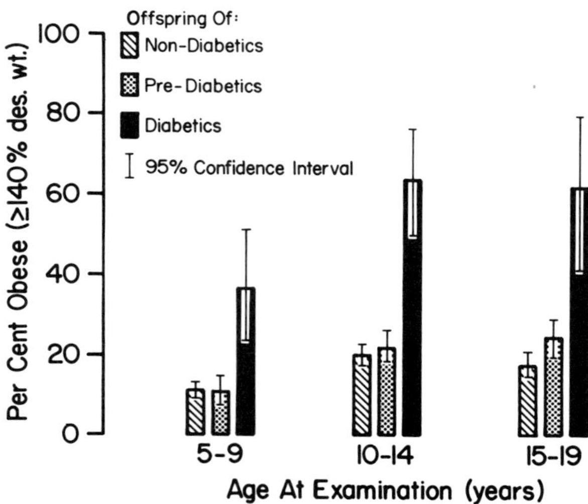

FIGURE 11.1. Prevalence of obesity among offspring of Pima Indians, according to age at examination and maternal status with respect to diabetes during gestation. (Reprinted by permission of the New England Journal of Medicine 308:242–245, 1983.)

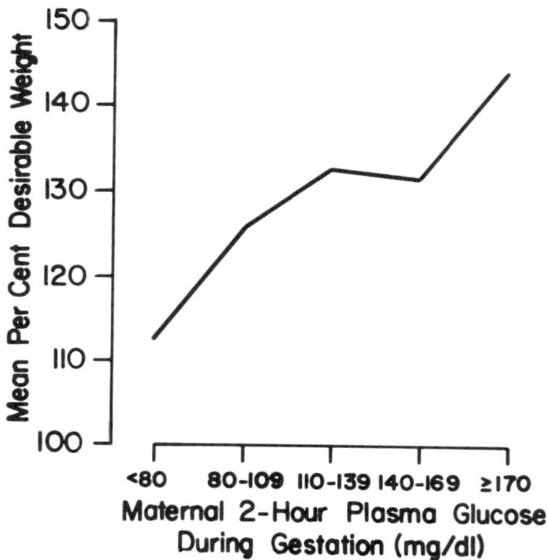

FIGURE 11.2. Mean percent of desirable weight for height in offspring at 15 to 19 years of age according to third-trimester maternal plasma glucose concentration among women without previously known diabetes. Glucose was drawn two hours after the ingestion of 75 g of carbohydrate during the third trimester of pregnancy.

data also suggest that the macrosomia associated with the newborn infant of the diabetic mother has different determinants than the obesity in later life.

Effect of Diabetes Control on Infant Obesity

Theoretically, control of maternal hyperglycemia should decrease both infantile macrosomia and long-term obesity of offspring of diabetic women. The effect of rigid blood glucose control during pregnancy on the offspring of the diabetic women has been evaluated (29,50–52). Infants whose mothers had well-controlled diabetes were not significantly different from offspring of nondiabetic women in birth weight. Infants of mothers with vascular complications had lower mean body weight. Infants of diabetic women who were examined at age 1 month were similar in length, weight, and skinfold thickness to infants of nondiabetic women. Another study among diabetic women (53) found no correlation between blood glucose control, assessed by the mean glucose concentration during the 2-week period prior to delivery, and infant birth weight. A comparison with the birth weight of infants of nondiabetic mothers was not reported. Among Pima Indian women without previously diagnosed diabetes, the prevalence of high infant birth weight appeared to be almost linearly related to maternal plasma glucose concentration measured during the third trimester (54).

Insulin Concentrations in the Offspring of Diabetic Mothers

Fetuses and Infants

Infant obesity may be a reflection of the effects of maternal glucose metabolism on the infant's metabolism (55,56). A more direct method of evaluating the relationship of maternal and infant metabolism is the measurement of the infant's plasma glucose and insulin concentrations. The intrauterine environment is thought to affect pancreatic function, which in turn affects fetal growth.

Infants of diabetic mothers have been shown to have higher insulin and C-peptide concentrations in cord blood and during the first few days of life than do controls (57–59). The C-peptide concentrations in the infants have been directly correlated with the severity of maternal diabetes and maternal glucose concentration. Similarly, in the fetus of the diabetic woman, the pancreas has been shown to contain more extractable insulin than in the fetuses of controls (60). In their studies of infants of diabetic women, Freinkel and his co-workers (61) have found that infants with accelerated somatic growth had higher concentrations of amniotic fluid insulin at 34 to 36 weeks gestation than did infants with normal growth patterns. Since amniotic fluid insulin is of fetal origin, this indicates that the fetal islets were already secreting excessive amounts of insulin.

Children and Adults

Amendt et al (62) compared insulin levels of children of insulin-dependent diabetic women with those of children of nondiabetic women. At 5 to 15 years of age, the highest insulin concentrations were in the offspring of mothers who had had the poorest glucose tolerance during pregnancy.

Several investigators (63–67) have examined the insulin response of the adult offspring of diabetic parents and the results have been inconclusive. Some investigators found the insulin response to be increased, some decreased, and others the same as in offspring with nondiabetic parents, but the results were obscured by many uncontrolled factors. Serum insulin concentrations are affected by hepatic metabolism, and therefore C-peptide may be a more accurate method of assessing pancreatic insulin production. Preliminary studies of C-peptide concentrations in the offspring of diabetic subjects also gave variable results. A group of adult offspring of two non-insulin-dependent diabetic parents had lower C-peptide concentrations than did a group of controls, but the insulin concentrations were variable. Both obese and nonobese offspring consistently had elevated insulin to C-peptide ratios, suggesting decreased hepatic metabolism of insulin (63). Also examined were young adult, nondiabetic offspring of patients with maturity-onset diabetes of the young, a disease with an autosomal dominant pattern of inheritance. These offspring were matched with controls for age, sex, and weight. Insulin concentrations were lower than those of controls in the obese, but not in the nonobese, offspring. The C-peptide concentrations were also lower than those of the controls in the obese group; but in the nonobese group, this was seen only in the fasting and one-half hour samples of an oral glucose tolerance test (64). Jackson et al (65) found that normal offspring of diabetic parents had higher fasting insulin concentrations than normal offspring of nondiabetic parents.

In contrast, Bonora et al (66) examined insulin secretion and disposal in a small number of adult offspring of couples with type II diabetes. Insulin and C-peptide concentrations and C-peptide to insulin ratios were not different from those of matched controls.

Abbott et al (68) examined a small number of 7 to 11-year-old offspring of prediabetic, diabetic, and nondiabetic Pima women. They found no statistically significant difference in fasting or stimulated insulin concentrations between the groups.

Elevated serum insulin concentrations so often present at birth in the offspring of diabetic women may result in hypoglycemia (57,58). Islet cell abnormalities, including hyperplasia and hypertrophy, remain after this transient hyperinsulinemia has resolved so that in offspring of diabetic women, islets make up more than three times as much of the pancreas as in offspring of nondiabetic mothers (69). If hypertrophy and hyperplasia of the islets persist, hyperinsulinemia and insulin resistance later in life may lead to the development of glucose intolerance and frank diabetes.

Glucose Tolerance in the Offspring of Diabetic Women

Heredity plays an important role in the development of diabetes, and there are numerous reports of high rates of diabetes in the offspring of people with diabetes (37,70–80). The potential effects of the intrauterine environment must be considered in the context of the genetic background, and these may be different in the offspring of women with type I than they are in the offspring of women with type II diabetes.

The diabetic intrauterine environment has been found to have a striking effect on glucose tolerance in the offspring of Pima Indians, a population with a very high prevalence of type II diabetes (81). Diabetes had a much higher prevalence (82,83) and incidence (84) in offspring of women who developed diabetes before pregnancy than in offspring of women who developed diabetes after the pregnancy or did not develop diabetes. The mean glucose concentration was also higher among the nondiabetic offspring of diabetic women than among the nondiabetic offspring of the other two groups of mothers (82). Among offspring of nondiabetic women, there is an association between the two-hour plasma glucose concentration of the mother during the third trimester and the offspring's glucose at age 15 to 19 years (Figure 11.3). Offspring of women who had glucose concentrations below the levels that would be diagnostic of diabetes during the nonpregnant state (85) have a mean glucose concentration that is almost as high as that of the offspring of diabetic women. These relationships do not appear affected by the age of onset of maternal diabetes, the father's diabetes status (86), or the child's degree of obesity (87).

Warram et al (88) pointed out that if the developing fetus were vulnerable to the lethal effects of the mother's diabetes and succumbed in utero, the effects of the intrauterine environment on the offspring would obscure the effects of inherited factors. However, if genetic factors predominate, glucose intolerance should occur at least as often in the offspring of a father with type I diabetes as in the offspring of a diabetic mother. Indeed, two studies have found lower rates of type I diabetes among offspring of diabetic mothers than of diabetic fathers (79,80). However, these results must be considered in light of the above possibility, i.e., a negative maternal diabetic influence in utero might result in selective loss of fetuses of diabetic mothers. Additionally, fetuses who are genetically susceptible to type I diabetes may be more susceptible to the lethal effects of the diabetic intrauterine environment and not survive long enough for diabetes to become manifest.

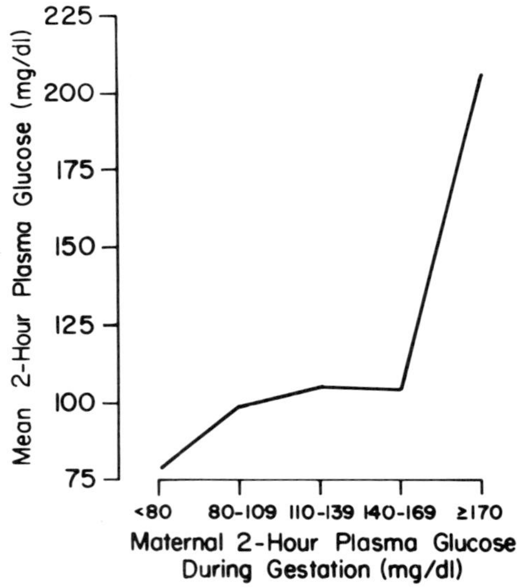

FIGURE 11.3. Mean two-hour postload plasma glucose concentration in offspring at 15 to 19 years of age according to third-trimester maternal plasma glucose of women without previously known diabetes.

Future Directions

Great strides have been made in the treatment of diabetes in general and the treatment of the pregnant diabetic woman in particular. Strict control of the diabetes, even if only during the latter part of pregnancy, has proved effective in reducing the incidence of perinatal morbidity and mortality in the newborn (50,89–92) as well as in decreasing the morbidity for the mother (50,91,93,94). Strict diabetes control prior to, as well as throughout, the pregnancy has been shown to reduce the incidence of congenital malformations (95), a lifelong complication for the offspring of diabetic women, which has not been dealt with in this chapter. But the work is far from finished. Glucose control during pregnancy needs to be better defined and quantified. Comparison of the offspring of women defined as prediabetic with the offspring of diabetic women will help differentiate genetic from intrauterine influences on the fetus. There is, as yet, no direct evidence that even the tightest control during the pregnancy will result in a long-term reduction in the rate of obesity and of diabetes in the offspring. However, there is some very compelling indirect evidence. Strict control of calorie intake during pregnancy and during the first year of life appears to prevent excessive fat accumulation during that period (96), and a low maternal calorie intake during the third trimester of pregnancy may be associated with lower rates of obesity in young adult men (97). Other evidence suggests that low calorie intake during pregnancy and early infancy may reduce the prevalence of diabetes as well (98,99). However, long term follow-up of the offspring of the well-controlled pregnancies is necessary. Hopefully, the optimal treatment of the mother during pregnancy will prove to be the optimal treatment not only for mother and newborn, but for the offspring in the long run as well. If control could be maximized to the extent that the fetus no longer recognizes that its mother has diabetes, then the treatment of the mother during the pregnancy, by preventing hyperinsulinemia in perinatal life, may become the first step in the prevention of obesity and diabetes in the offspring.

References

1. Martin RJ, Ramsay T, Hausman GJ (1984) Adipocyte development. Pediatr Ann 13:448–453.
2. Ashwell M (1985) The use of the adipose tissue transplantation technique to demonstrate that abnormalities in the adipose tissue metabolism of genetically obese mice are due to extrinsic rather than intrinsic factors. Int J Obes 9[suppl 1]:77–82.
3. Nixon T, Green H (1984) Contribution of growth hormone to the adipogenic activity of serum. Endocrinology 114:527–532.
4. Roncari DAK, Van RLR (1978) Promotion of human adipocyte precursor replication by 17 β-estradiol in culture. J Clin Invest 62:503–508.

5. Hayashi I, Nixon T, Morikawa M, Green H (1981) Adipogenic and anti-adipogenic factors in the pituitary and other organs. Proc Natl Acad Sci USA 78:3969–3972.
6. Vannier C, Gaillard D, Grimaldi P, Amri E-Z, Djian P, Cermolacce C, Forest C, Etienne J, Negrel R, Ailhaud G (1985) Adipose conversion of ob17 cells and hormone-related events. Int J Obes 9[Suppl 1]:41–53.
7. Green H, Kehinde O (1975) An established preadipose cell line and its differentiation in culture II. Factors affecting the adipose conversion. Cell 5:19–27.
8. Kuri-Harcuch W, Carrera-de la Torre B, Arkuch-Kuri S, Beltran-Langarica A (1985) Human adipogenic serum activity increases during pregnancy. Int J Obes 9:299–306.
9. Hausman GJ, Campion DR, Martin RJ (1980) Search for the adipocyte precursor cell and factors that promote its differentiation. J Lipid Res 21:657–670.
10. Bonnet FP, Rocour-Brumioul D (1981) Normal growth of human adipose tissue, in Bonnet FP (ed): Adipose Tissue in Childhood. CRC Press, Boca Raton, FL, pp 81–107.
11. Enzi G, Inelmen M, Cordioli G, Baritussio A (1976) Fat cell size, weight and number in children in relation to anthropometric and metabolic parameters, in Lazon Z, Dickerman Z (eds): Pediatric and Adolescent Endocrinology, vol 1: The Adipose Child. S Karger, Basel, pp 119–129.
12. Häger A (1981) Adipose tissue cellularity in childhood in relation to the development of obesity. Br Med Bull 37:287–290.
13. Enzi G, Inelmen EM, Caretta F, Rubaltelli F, Grella P, Baritussio A (1980) Adipose tissue development "in utero." Relationships between some nutritional and hormonal factors and body fat mass enlargement in newborns. Diabetologia 18:135–140.
14. Hirsch J, Knittle JL (1970) Cellularity of obese and nonobese human adipose tissue. Fed Proc 29:1516–1521.
15. Knittle JL, Timmers K, Ginsberg-Fellner F, Brown RE, Katz DP (1979) The growth of adipose tissue in children and adolescents. Cross-sectional and longitudinal studies of adipose cell number and size. J Clin Invest 63:239–246.
16. Dauncey MJ, Gairdner D (1975) Size of adipose cells in infancy. Arch Dis Child 50:286–290.
17. Stunkard AJ, Sørensen TIA, Hanis C, Teasdale TW, Chakraborty R, Schull WJ, Schulsinger F (1986) An adoption study of Human Obesity. N Engl J Med 314:193–198.
18. Biron P, Mongeau J-G, Bertrand D (1977) Familial resemblance of body weight and weight/height in 374 homes with adopted children. J Pediatr 91:555–558.
19. Shenker IR, Fisichelli V, Lang J (1974) Weight differences between foster infants of overweight and nonoverweight foster mothers. J Pediatr 84:715–719.
20. Poehlman ET, Tremblay A, Després J-P, Fontaine E, Pérusse L, Thériault G, Bouchard C (1986) Genotype-controlled changes in body composition and fat morphology following overfeeding in twins. Am J Clin Nutr 43:723–731.
21. Börjeson M (1976) The aetiology of obesity in children. A study of 101 twin pairs. Acta Paediatr Scand 65:279–287.

22. Ginsberg-Fellner F (1981) Growth of adipose tissue in infants, children and adolescents: variations in growth disorders. Int J Obes 5:605–611.
23. Fisch RO, Bilek MK, Ulstrom R (1975) Obesity and leanness at birth and their relationship to body habitus in later childhood. Pediatrics 56:521–528.
24. Harrison GG, Udall JN, Morrow G (1980) Maternal obesity, weight gain in pregnancy, and infant birth weight. Am J Obstet Gynecol 136:411–412.
25. Murata Y, Martin CB (1973) Growth of the biparietal diameter of the fetal head in diabetic pregnancy. Am J Obstet Gynecol 115:252–256.
26. Kuhns LR, Berger PE, Roloff DW, Poznanski AK, Holt JF (1974) Fat thickness in the newborn infant of a diabetic mother. Radiology 111:665–671.
27. Enzi G, Inelmen EM, Caretta F, Villani F, Zanardo V, DeBiasi F (1980) Development of adipose tissue in newborns of gestational-diabetic and insulin-dependent diabetic mothers. Diabetes 29:100–104.
28. Cardell BS (1953) The infants of diabetic mothers. A morphological study. J Obstet Gynaecol Br Emp 60:834–853.
29. Wurster PA, Kochenour NK, Thomas MR (1984) Infant adiposity and maternal energy consumption in well-controlled diabetics. J Am Coll Nutr 3:75–83.
30. Heald FP, Hollander RJ (1965) The relationship between obesity in adolescence and early growth. J Pediatr 67:35–38.
31. Dine MS, Gartside PS, Glueck CJ, Rheines L, Greene G, Khoury P (1979) Where do the heaviest children come from? A prospective study of white children from birth to 5 years of age. Pediatrics 63:1–7.
32. Björntorp P, Enzi G, Karlsson K, Krotkiewski M, Sjöström L, Smith U (1974) The effect of maternal diabetes on adipose tissue cellularity in man and rat. Diabetologia 10:205–209.
33. Harrison GG, White M, Goldsby JB (1977) Relationship of birthweight to risk of infantile obesity. Pediatr Res 11:436.
34. Whitelaw A (1977) Subcutaneous fat in newborn infants of diabetic mothers: An indication of quality of diabetic control. Lancet 1:15–18.
35. Ginsberg-Fellner F, Knittle JL (1971) Maternal diabetes as a factor in the development of childhood obesity. Soc Ped Res 41:197.
36. Abbott WGH, Thuillez P, Howard BV, Bennett PH, Salans LB, Cushman SW, Reaven GM, Foley JE (1986) Body composition, adipocyte size, free fatty acid concentration, and glucose tolerance in children of diabetic pregnancies. Diabetes 35:1077–1080.
37. White P, Koshy P, Duckers J (1953) The management of pregnancy complicating diabetes and of children of diabetic mothers. Med Clin North Am 39:1481–1496.
38. Breidahl HD (1966) The growth and development of children born to mothers with diabetes. Med J Aust 1:268–270.
39. Adler P, Fett KD, Bohátka L (1977) The influence of maternal diabetes on dental development of the non-diabetic offspring in the stage of transitional dentition. Acta Paediatr Acad Sci Hung 18:181–195.
40. Fredrikson H, Hagbard L, Olow I, Reinand R (1957) Follow-up investigation of children of diabetic mothers. Nord Med 57:669–671.
41. Weitz R, Laron Z, (1976) Height and weight of children born to mothers with diabetes mellitus. Isr J Med Sci 12:195–198.
42. Farquhar JW (1959) The child of the diabetic woman. Arch Dis Child 34:76–96.

43. Farquhar JW (1969) Prognosis for babies born to diabetic mothers in Edinburgh. Arch Dis Child 44:36–47.
44. Shah MPK, Farquhar JW (1975) Children of diabetic mothers-subsequent weight, in Camerini-Davalos RA, Cole HS (eds): Early Diabetes in Early Life. Academic Press, New York, pp 587–608.
45. Hagbard L, Olow I, Reinand T (1959) A follow-up study of 514 children of diabetic mothers. Acta Paediatr 48:184–197.
46. Vohr BR, Lipsitt LP, Oh W (1980) Somatic growth of children of diabetic mothers with reference to birth size. J Pediatr 97:196–199.
47. Pettitt DJ, Baird HR, Aleck KA, Bennett PH, Knowler WC (1983) Excessive obesity in offspring of Pima Indian women with diabetes during pregnancy. N Engl J Med 308:242–245.
48. Pettitt DJ, Bennett PH, Knowler WC, Baird HR, Aleck KA (1985) Gestational diabetes mellitus and impaired glucose tolerance during pregnancy. Long-term effects on obesity and glucose tolerance in the offspring. Diabetes 34:119–122.
49. Pettitt DJ, Knowler WC, Bennett PH, Aleck KA, Baird HR (1987) Obesity in offspring of diabetic Pima Indian women despite normal birth weight. Diabetes Care 10:76–80.
50. Jovanovic L, Druzin M, Peterson CM (1981) Effect of Euglycemia on the outcome of pregnancy in insulin-dependent diabetic women as compared with normal control subjects. Am J Med 71:921–927.
51. Gyves MT, Rodman HM, Little AB, Fanaroff AA, Merkatz IR (1977) A modern approach to management of pregnant diabetics: A two-year analysis of perinatal outcomes. Am J Obstet Gynecol 128:606–616.
52. Khojandi M, Tsai AY-M, Tyson JE (1974) Gestational diabetes: The dilemma of delivery. Obstet Gynecol 43:1–6.
53. Karlsson K, Kjellmer I (1972) The outcome of diabetic pregnancies in relation to the mother's blood sugar level. Am J Obstet Gynecol 112:213–220.
54. Pettitt DJ, Knowler WC, Baird HR, Bennett PH (1980) Gestational diabetes: Infant and maternal complications of pregnancy in relation to third-trimester glucose tolerance in the Pima Indians. Diabetes Care 3:458–464.
55. Obenshain SS, Adam PAJ, King KC, Teramo K, Raivio KO, Räihä N, Schwartz R (1970) Human fetal insulin response to sustained maternal hyperglycemia. N Engl J Med 283:566–570.
56. Pedersen J, Osler M (1961) Hyperglycemia as the cause of characteristic features of the foetus and newborn of diabetic mothers. Dan Med Bull 8:78–83.
57. Stimmler L, Brazie JV, O'Brien D (1964) Plasma-insulin levels in the newborn infants of normal and diabetic mothers. Lancet 1:137–138.
58. Sosenko IR, Kitzmiller JL, Loo SW, Blix P, Rubenstein AH, Gabbay KH (1979) The infant of the diabetic mother. Correlation of increased cord C-peptide levels with macrosomia and hypoglycemia. N Engl J Med 301:859–862.
59. Heding LG, Persson B, Stangenberg M (1980) B-cell function in newborn infants of diabetic mothers. Diabetologia 19:427–432.
60. Steinke J, Driscoll SG (1965) The extractable insulin content of pancreas from fetuses and infants of diabetic and control mothers. Diabetes 14:573–578.
61. Freinkel N (1980) Banting Lecture 1980. Of pregnancy and progeny. Diabetes 29:1023–1035.

62. Amendt P, Michaelis D, Hildmann W (1976) Clinical and metabolic studies in children of diabetic mothers. Endokrinology 67:351–361.
63. Snehalatha C, Mohan V, Ramachandran A, Jayashree R, Viswanathan M (1984) Pancreatic beta cell function in offspring of conjugal diabetic parents. Assessment by IRI and C-peptide ratio. Horm Metab Res [Suppl]16:142–144.
64. Mohan V, Snehalatha C, Ramachandran A, Viswanathan M (1986) Abnormalities in insulin secretion in healthy offspring of Indian patients with maturity-onset diabetes of the young. Diabetes Care 9:53–56.
65. Jackson WPU, van Mieghem W, Keller P (1972) Insulin excess as the initial lesion in diabetes. Lancet 1:1040–1044.
66. Bonora E, Zavaroni I, Bruschi F, Alpi O, Pezzarossa A, Dall'Aglio E, Coscelli C, Butturini U (1984) Evidence for unimpaired pancreatic secretion and hepatic removal of insulin in healthy offspring of type 2 (noninsulin-dependent) diabetic couples. Horm Res 20:138–142.
67. Persson B, Gentz J, Möller E (1984) Follow-up of children of insulin dependent (Type I) and gestational diabetic mothers. Growth pattern, glucose tolerance, insulin response, and HLA types. Acta Paediatr Scand 73:778–784.
68. Abbott WG, Foley JE (1985) Neither gestational diabetes nor a positive family history of diabetes influences body composition, adipocyte size or insulin or glucose concentrations. Diabetes 34[Suppl 1]:125A.
69. Naeye RL (1965) Infants of diabetic mothers: A quantitative, morphologic study. Pediatrics 35:980–988.
70. White P (1960) The Banting Memorial Lecture 1960. Childhood diabetes. Its course, and influence on the second and third generations. Diabetes 9:345–355.
71. Simpson NE (1968) Diabetes in the families of diabetics. Can Med Assoc J 98:427–432.
72. Simpson NE (1969) Heritabilities of liability to diabetes when sex and age at onset are considered. Ann Hum Genet [Lond] 32:283–303.
73. Yssing M (1975) Long-term prognosis of children born to mothers diabetic when pregnant, in Camerini-Davalos RA, Cole HS (eds): Early Diabetes in Early Life. Academic Press, New York, pp 575–586.
74. Bibergeil H, Godel E, Amendt P (1975) Diabetes and pregnancy: Early and late prognosis of children of diabetic mothers, in Camerini-Davalos RA, Cole HS (eds): Early Diabetes in Early Life. Academic Press, New York, pp 427–434.
75. Lee ET, Anderson PS, Bryan J, Bahr C, Coniglione T, Cleves M (1985) Diabetes, parental diabetes, and obesity in Oklahoma Indians. Diabetes Care 8:107–113.
76. Knowler WC, Pettitt DJ, Savage PJ, Bennett PH (1981) Diabetes incidence in Pima Indians: Contributions of obesity and parental diabetes. Am J Epidem 113:144–156.
77. Köbberling J, Brüggeboes B (1980) Prevalence of diabetes among children of insulin-dependent diabetic mothers. Diabetologia 18:459–462.
78. Radder JK, Terpstra J (1975) The incidence of diabetes mellitus in the offspring of diabetic couples. Investigation based on the oral glucose tolerance test. Diabetologia 11:135–138.
79. Wagener DK, Sacks JM, LaPorte RE, MacGregor JM (1982) The Pittsburgh

study of insulin-dependent diabetes mellitus. Risk for diabetes among relatives of IDDM. Diabetes 31:136–144.

80. Dahlquist G, Blom L, Holmgren G, Hägglöf B, Larsson Y, Sterky G, Wall S (1985) The epidemiology of diabetes in Swedish children 0–14 years—a six-year prospective study. Diabetologia 28:801–808.

81. Knowler WC, Bennett PH, Hamman RF, Miller M (1978) Diabetes incidence and prevalence in Pima Indians: A 19-fold greater incidence than in Rochester, Minnesota. Am J Epidem 108:497–505.

82. Pettitt DJ, Baird HR, Aleck KA, Knowler WC (1982) Diabetes mellitus in children following maternal diabetes during gestation. Diabetes 31[Suppl 2]:66A.

83. Pettitt DJ (1986) The long-range impact of diabetes during pregnancy: The Pima Indian experience. International Diabetes Federation Bull 31:70–71.

84. Pettitt DJ, Bennett PH. Long-term outcome of infants of diabetic mothers, in Reece EA, Coustan D, Hobbins JC (eds): Diabetes in Pregnancy: Principles and Practice. Churchill Livingstone, New York (in press).

85. WHO Study Group (1985) Diabetes mellitus. World Health Organization Technical Report Series 727. World Health Organization, Geneva.

86. Pettitt D, Baird H, Carraher M, Knowler W (1984) Genetic and intrauterine environmental effects in transmission of diabetes mellitus. Am J Epidem 120:477.

87. Pettitt DJ, Bennett PH, Everhart J, Kunzelman CL, Knowler WC (1985) High plasma glucose concentration in normal weight offspring of diabetic women. Diabetes Res Clin Pract 1[Suppl 1]:S445.

88. Warram JH, Krolewski AS, Gottlieb MS, Kahn CR (1984) Differences in risk of insulin-dependent diabetes in offspring of diabetic mothers and diabetic fathers. N Engl J Med 311:149–152.

89. Adashi EY, Pinto H, Tyson JE (1979) Impact of maternal euglycemia on fetal outcome in diabetic pregnancy. Am J Obstet Gynecol 133:268–274.

90. Coustan DR, Berkowitz RL, Hobbins JC (1980) Tight metabolic control of overt diabetes in pregnancy. Am J Med 68:845–852.

91. Coustan DR, Imarah J (1984) Prophylactic insulin treatment of gestational diabetes reduces the incidence of macrosomia, operative delivery, and birth trauma. Am J Obstet Gynecol 150:836–842.

92. Reller MD, Tsang RC, Meyer RA, Braun CP (1985) Relationship of prospective diabetes control in pregnancy to neonatal cardiorespiratory function. J Pediatr 106:86–90.

93. Jervell J, Moe N, Skjæraasen J, Blystad W, Egge K (1979) Diabetes mellitus and pregnancy—Management and results at Rikshospitalet, Oslo, 1970–1977. Diabetologia 16:151–155.

94. Jervell J, Stokke KT, Moe N, Haugen HN, Vidnes J (1979) Metabolic profiles in closely controlled diabetic pregnancies during the third trimester. Diabetologia 16:229–233.

95. Fuhrmann K, Reiher H, Semmler K, Fischer F, Fischer M, Glöckner E (1983) Prevention of congenital malformations in infants of insulin-dependent diabetic mothers. Diabetes Care 6:219–223.

96. Enzi G, Inelmen EM, Rubaltelli FF, Zanardo V, Favaretto L (1982) Postnatal development of adipose tissue in normal children on strictly controlled calorie intake. Metabolism 31:1029–1034.

97. Ravelli G-P, Stein ZA, Susser MW (1976) Obesity in young men after famine exposure in utero and early infancy. N Engl J Med 195:349–353.
98. Dörner G, Mohnike A, Thoelke H (1984) Further evidence for the dependence of diabetes prevalence on nutrition in perinatal life. Exp Clin Endocrinol 84:129–133.
99. Dörner G, Steindel E, Thoelke H, Schliack V (1984) Evidence for decreasing prevalence of diabetes mellitus in childhood apparently produced by prevention of hyperinsulinism in the foetus and newborn. Exp Clin Endocrinol 84:134–142.

Index

Oral hypoglycemic agents (*see* Hypoglycemic agents, oral)

P

Pancreas, fetal (*see* Fetal pancreas)

Perinatal mortality and morbidity (*see* Gestational diabetes, perinatal mortality and morbidity associated with)

Phenformin, 62, 67, 68

Phosphatidylglycerol, 159–160

Placenta
  amino acid transport across, 129
  function of, assessment of, 116, 142
  glucagon receptors of, 34
  glucose transport across, 16, 129
  growth hormone/growth factors produced by, 34, 36
  growth hormone receptors of, 34
  insufficiency of, diabetes-induced, 116
  insulin receptors of, 34
  insulin transport across, 20, 36, 129
  lactogen receptors of, 34, 129
  morphologic changes of, 15–16
    blood flow, 15
    cystic vacuoles, 15
    fibrin deposits, 15
    glycogen content, 15
    lipid content, 15
  somatomedin production of, 36
  thyroid disorder drug transport across, 95–96
  vascular disease and, 156

Polyhydramnios, 139

Pregestational diabetes
  fetal effects of, 136–138
    intrauterine death, 136
    macrosomia, 138
    malformations, 136–137
    small-for-gestational age size, 134
  maternal effects of, 135–136
    diabetic ketoacidosis, 135
    hypoglycemia, 135
    nephropathy, 136
    retinopathy, 136
  maternal mortality, 134

neonatal effects, 138–139
    hyperbilirubinemia, 139
    hypoglycemia, 138–139
    respiratory distress syndrome, 138
  oral hypoglycemic drug therapy, effect of, 63–65
  perinatal mortality, 134
  premature delivery and, 134–135

Pregnancy
  anatomic changes during, 101–102
  blood glucose levels during, 131–133
  blood volume during, 102
  cardiac output during, 102
  connective tissue changes during, 101
  diabetes mellitus after, 60, 130, 132
    oral glucose tolerance test of, 133
    retinopathy of, 136
  diabetes mellitus before (*see* Pregestational diabetes)
  diabetic (*see* Gestational diabetes)
  exercise during, effects of (*see* Exercise)
  glycosuria of, 131
  heart rate during, 102
  hemodynamic changes during, 102
  insulin requirements during, 133
  insulin resistance, 130
  metabolic adaptations of, 129–130
  metabolic control during, 133
  nutritional requirements during, 104
  orthopedic problems of, 108
  vertebral column during, changes in, 102

Premature delivery
  complications of, 115
  fetal surveillance and, 142
  hyperbilirubinemia and, 139
  hypocalcemia and, 163
  indications for, 136
  induced labor, 134
  maternal mortality, 134
  neonatal effects of, 138–139
  perinatal mortality, 134–135

Progesterone, 129

Prolactin, 129